Managing the
Medical Arms Race

Managing the Medical Arms Race

Public Policy and Medical Device Innovation

SUSAN BARTLETT FOOTE

UNIVERSITY OF CALIFORNIA PRESS
Berkeley   Los Angeles   Oxford

University of California Press
Berkeley and Los Angeles, California

University of California Press, Ltd.
Oxford, England

© 1992 by
The Regents of the University of California

Library of Congress Cataloging-in-Publication Data

Foote, Susan Bartlett.
Managing the medical arms race : public policy and medical device
innovation / Susan Bartlett Foote.
p.   cm.
Includes bibliographical references and index.
ISBN 0-520-07591-9 (cloth : alk. paper)
1. Medical instruments and apparatus industry—Government policy.
[1. Diffusion of Innovation. 2. Equipment and Supplies—standards—
United States. 3. Public Policy—United States.] I. Title.
[DNLM: W 26 F689m]
HD994.U52F66   1992
338.4'7681761'0973—dc20
DNLM/DLC
for Library of Congress   91-843
CIP

Printed in the United States of America

9 8 7 6 5 4 3 2 1

To my children,
Rebecca and Benjamin

Contents

Tables and Figures

Preface

This book provides a comprehensive look at the wide range of public policies that affect innovation in the medical device industry. It is a case study of the interaction between technology and policy—the relationship between private industry and government institutions. It is a tale that appeals to our most optimistic views about the ability of American know-how to diminish pain and suffering. It is also the story of technological failures and disappointments, a story that reveals the strengths and weaknesses of America's public and private institutions. Because we all live and will probably die surrounded by medical devices, the consequences of this interaction between government and business affect the health care choices that we as patients will have in the future.

The products of the medical device industry are probably more familiar to readers than the term *medical device* might convey. There is considerable popular interest in such innovations as the controversial intrauterine device (IUD), lithotripsy machines that crush kidney stones without surgery, angioplasty performed with lasers that remove plaque deposits from coronary arteries, and life-support systems for premature infants, to name only a few of the over 3,500 different products on the market.

Despite the importance of medical device innovations, the interrelationship of the industry to government policy is neither well studied nor well understood. Indeed, knowledge of the device industry has not expanded as rapidly as its relative importance to health care. There are good and useful data and analyses, but they are scattered across many fields or cover only a limited amount of the story told here. There is extensive literature on innovation, but it often diminishes or ignores the impact of public policy.[1] There are excellent studies of particular public institutions, upon which I have relied, but they do not focus exclusively on medical devices.[2] There are also excellent case studies of individual medical device technologies, including kidney dialysis, artificial organs, and the artificial heart.[3]

Much of the groundwork for this book has been laid by the technical studies of the Office of Technology Assessment, a research division of the U.S. Congress.[4] Health policy analysts have examined important aspects of the medical device industry, and my debt to them is gratefully acknowledged.[5] The extensive citations throughout this book testify to the serious scholarship that is relevant to an understanding of the issues addressed.

My aim is to provide a more comprehensive overview of the interaction of public policy and innovation than is currently available. I have been interested in medical device technology and policy for well over a decade, and sections of this book draw on my previous work.[6] I hope to do for medical devices what Paul Starr accomplished for the medical profession, Charles Rosenberg and Rosemary Stevens have done for hospitals, and Henry Grabowski has contributed to our understanding of the pharmaceutical industry.[7] A formidable task indeed!

The discussion is accessible to all readers interested in medical technology and health policy regardless of training or expertise. Too often, the temptation among academics is to speak only to their own kind, communicating in the shorthand of their scholarly disciplines. Such a self-protective ploy is not possible here because of the wide range of issues and the breadth of the potential audience. The challenge, which I hope has been met, is to tell the story without cloaking the message in unnecessary technical jargon.

This book is also designed to add to the more specialized knowledge of experts. These readers may benefit from exposure to areas of policy that their own work does not address. For example, the analyst who spends his days implementing Medicare policy at the Health Care Financing Administration in Washington (HCFA) may not realize the relevance of product liability or federal regulation to the very innovations he assesses for payment or coverage purposes. The same is true for the physician who may know much about certain medical devices but little about the role of government in determining their cost and availability and for the product manager who may see the government only as a barrier to her marketing plan.

Students of business-government relations will find that the medical device industry provides an interesting case study of policy proliferation problems that affect other sectors of the economy as well. Extensive chapter references should help all readers pursue particular issues in greater depth.

In writing this book, I personally encountered the negative and the positive aspects of medical devices. I brought the manuscript along when I took my mother for radiation treatments during her valiant, but losing, battle with lung cancer. There seemed no end to the technological fixes that offered false hopes and that only prolonged pain and suffering. I saw firsthand the role of technology as a substitute for the caring side of medicine. On a more optimistic note, I brought this manuscript to the hospital when I underwent two operations on my own back. These procedures were successful in large part because of the advanced state of diagnostic imaging and the whole range of technological innovations in surgical technique. While this form of field research is one I do not care to repeat, I acquired new respect for these costly, yet effective and beneficial, technological advances.

Of course, my exposure to medical technology is not unique. All of us have felt the impact of the health care system and its technology on ourselves and our families. The innovations and the institutions discussed in this book inevitably touch us all.

No book is complete without acknowledgments. I am indebted to colleagues in the Business and Public Policy Group at the Walter A. Haas School of Business at the University of California, Berkeley, including Budd Cheit, Edwin Epstein, Robert Harris, David Irons, David Mowery, Christine Rosen, and David Vogel, who commented on various drafts. Others at Berkeley provided useful critique and support, including Sally Fairfax, Judy Gruber, Charles O'Reilly, and Franklin Zimring. Dr. Stephen Bongard recently of the Institute of Medicine and Dr. Peter Budetti of the George Washington University School of Medicine shared their expertise and experiences at various stages of this project.

Students of law and business at Berkeley, including Richard S. Taylor, Ann R. Shulman, Kenneth Koput, Dr. David Okuji, Dr. Michael J. Sterns, Brian Shaffer, and Emerson Tiller, provided able research assistance, and the Harris Trust at the Institute for

Governmental Studies at Berkeley and the Program in Business and Social Policy supplied funds for their support. I am also grateful to the Institute of Medicine at the National Academy of Sciences, which provided forums for thoughtful analysis and debate of important health policy issues in which I was invited to participate. Serena Joe helped with typing the manuscript and Patricia Murphy provided meticulous word processing and editorial advice.

When the urge to abandon was strongest, I was encouraged by William Lowrance of The Rockefeller University, who believed in the idea and sustained me in the early stages. I am grateful to Robert Coleman, who could always make me laugh, and to Ed Freeman of the University of Virginia, who knew there was a story to be told.

During the 1990–1991 academic year, I was fortunate to have been selected as a Robert Wood Johnson Congressional Health Policy Fellow. I extend deep appreciation to Marion Ein Lewin, the director of the fellowship, and to the five other RWJ fellows who served as colleagues, teachers, and most of all as friends. I am especially indebted to Senator Dave Durenberger and his exceptional staff, who allowed me to participate in the Senate health policy process in the first session of the 102d Congress.

PART ONE
THE DIAGNOSIS

The machine itself makes no demands and holds
out no promises: it is the human spirit that makes
demands and keeps promises.

Lewis Mumford
Technics and Civilization

1

THE DIAGNOSTIC FRAMEWORK

The gains in technics are never registered automatically in society; they require equally adroit
inventions and adaptations in politics; and the
careless habit of attributing to mechanical improvements a direct role as instruments of culture and civilization puts a demand upon the
machine to which it cannot respond. . . .

No matter how completely technics relies upon
the objective procedures of the sciences, it does
not form an independent system, like the uni-
verse; it exists as an element in human culture
and it promises well or ill as the social groups that
exploit it promise well or ill. The machine itself
makes no demands and holds out no promises: it
is the human spirit that makes demands and
keeps promises.

Lewis Mumford
Technics and Civilization

THE PROBLEM

Medical devices, the "technics" of this book, pervade our experiences with health care throughout our lives—from fetal monitoring equipment and ultrasound imaging before birth to life-
support systems and even suicide machines when death is near.[1]
Medical care has become increasingly dependent on technology,
and medical devices are the epitome of the trend. The modern hospital is a wonderland of complicated machinery, and
the rhythmic beeping of heart monitors evokes a life-and-death
drama. Tens of thousands of Americans depend upon artificial
body parts for survival and to improve the quality of their lives—

from hips to intraocular lenses to heart pacemakers. Even doctors' offices are full of new devices. Physicians use lasers to remove cataracts without the need for hospitalization; ultrasound monitors take pictures of unborn babies. The allure of medical innovation is powerful, holding out the possibility of a perfect outcome, an amelioration of pain, a delay in our inexorable decline toward death.

Spending on medical devices reflects this trend. This multibillion dollar industry producing thousands of products may account for as much as 40 percent of the health care bill, which has grown to close to 12 percent of the gross national product.[2] (See figure 1.) The demand seems insatiable. We have come to expect a steady stream of new "miracles." Experts predict bloodless laser surgery in the near future and a genetic engineering revolution at the turn of the century. "At the current rate of innovation," an analyst recently projected, "by the year 2000 close to 100,000 new or enhanced medical devices will be introduced into the marketplace. Health care will be a $1.5 trillion industry."[3]

Demand is fueled by our belief in equitable access to medical care. When a medical innovation is considered beneficial, there is pressure to distribute its benefits to all who need it. News stories of people denied access to high-cost treatments because of their inability to pay generate public sympathy and, often, outrage. Until very recently, the ideal of the highest quality care for everyone has been rarely questioned, albeit unattained.

Medical technology is not without critics who challenge any unquestioning belief in its value. Some argue that in our love affair with technology we have sacrificed the caring, or service, side of medicine.[4] The public is also intolerant of technologies that cause harm. The dangers of the Dalkon Shield, an intrauterine device (IUD) that injured thousands of women, received widespread publicity. In a recent controversy, the government has charged that a medical device producer marketed heart valves it knew to be defectively designed, leaving thousands in daily fear that their implanted devices will fail and kill them.[5]

Some blame medical technology for the escalating costs of care as well. There is no question that some technology is expensive, but other products reduce costs through early diagnosis or

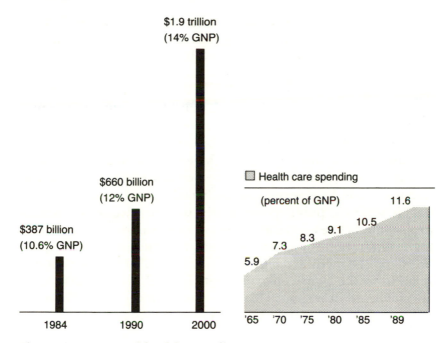

Figure 1. Forecasted health spending.
Sources: (a) M. S. Freeland et al., *Health Care Financing Review* 6 (Spring 1985): 1–20; and K. W. Tyson and J. C. Merrill, *Journal of Medical Education* 59 (1984): 773–81; (b) Health Care Financing Administration.

shorter hospital stays. Pressures to control costs have led to calls for elimination of wasteful or unnecessarily expensive equipment. Exposure of fraud in the cardiac pacemaker industry and of unnecessary implants of intraocular lenses lend credence to this charge.[6]

Even highly desirable technologies are controversial. There can be tension between providing access to expensive lifesaving devices to a few and more widespread access to lower-cost benefits to many. In a recent policy decision, Oregon medical officials declared that the Medicaid program, which serves the poor in that state, would no longer pay for liver transplants, a desirable high-cost, lifesaving technology, in order to use the funds to cover prenatal care for a larger number of low-income pregnant women. The state also recommended a priority list to determine which treatments would be covered under the program.[7] This is one example of the many explicit and implicit tradeoffs that are made as public and private budgets are stretched to the limit.

Medical device innovations—with lifesaving promises, potential risks, and often high price tags—are deeply embedded in the broad debates about health policy. The insatiable demand, fed by a profusion of new technologies and the profits they represent, has been called the medical arms race. Increasingly, government has been called upon to manage it.

This book explores the "adroit inventions and adaptations in politics" that have accompanied the profusion of medical devices in our society. As government has become inextricably linked to health services, public policies affecting medical devices have proliferated. These policies reflect diverse values and arise from many different institutions. Because of the pervasiveness of public policy, the medical device industry can only be understood in relation to the policy environment. Indeed, the industry grew and matured in response to public policy incentives. Those responses, in turn, brought new layers of public policy.

A medically related analogy will help to structure the discussion. Policy proliferation is analogous to polypharmacy, an increasingly familiar condition to the health care profession. Polypharmacy occurs when a patient takes a number of prescription drugs. Each prescription may have been given for a legitimate ailment, but the interactions between the drugs can harm the patient. Attentive doctors routinely request that patients put all their drugs in a brown paper bag and bring them in for review. The review evaluates what is known about the drugs and what is known about the particular patient. There may be new information about a drug product, and there may also be changes in the patient's underlying condition. A physician must look for possible interactions between the drugs. Some reactions may be previously unknown or unexpected; some predictable and even tolerable. Some may dissipate the efficacy of other prescriptions and require modifications of dosage, and some may be fatal.

This book provides a "brown-bag" review of all the policies that directly and indirectly affect the medical device industry. The industry is the patient; the present policies are the prescriptions to which the patient reacts and responds. The book begins the diagnosis by asking key questions: What is the impact of these multiple prescriptions on the patient? On the medical device industry? Are our prescriptions producing desirable outcomes without adverse and unexpected side effects? Is the result good health—in this case, meaningful innovation that is safe, efficacious, efficient, and cost effective? If not, what revisions in the treatment are appropriate? What is the patient's prognosis?

To answer these questions, we must take the patient's history, review each prescription to determine when and why it was offered, how it has changed over time, and how it relates to other prescriptions. After extensive review of these factors, the conclusion is mixed. It would, of course, be dramatic to report that government policy has destroyed device innovation; that is, the side effects are worse than the treatment. The reality is less definitive and more elusive. Until the 1990s, we have managed to muddle along, balancing myriad policy goals. Innovation flourished in the 1950s and 1960s because the dominant policies promoted both discovery of new products and their widespread distribution. Innovation has survived in the 1970s and 1980s despite safety and cost-control policies that inhibit innovation. The momentum of innovation was sustained in part because these policies were relatively unsuccessful in accomplishing their goals. Regulation was not fully implemented as intended, product liability had only sporadic effects on certain devices, and cost-containment strategies could not combat the pressure for distribution of benefits. If these policies had been successful, the industry would have been more adversely affected.

What does the future hold? We can expect renewed efforts to impose greater regulation and more effective cost controls in the 1990s. There is clear evidence of overdiffusion that government may try to control. As the marketplace attracts more equipment and as technicians and specialists arise to operate it, there can be supply-induced demand. In other words, if a facility has an MRI machine, it will find the patients necessary to operate the machine at a profit.

Policies to control supply costs can be on a collision course with the competing desire for more innovative devices. When public policies clash, there can be serious adverse reactions for innovation. The departure of most childhood vaccine producers in the wake of product liability suits and the impact of regulation and liability on innovation in contraceptive research and development have been well documented.[8] These cases represent potential adverse effects of public policy that we must seek to avoid with other devices.

Muddling through the 1990s will not be acceptable. If we allow the situation to drift, we could become passive observers of unwanted outcomes. However, prevention of harmful effects is possible. Reforms that affirmatively balance competing values while eliminating conflicts and redundancies are presented here. Incremental accommodations can relieve some of the stresses on the system. But we must recognize the limits of medical device technology to cure all ills and the limits of public policy to solve social problems. Indeed, wise policy must address the larger moral questions of how we want to live and how we want to die: difficult questions we tend to avoid.

Medical devices are sufficiently important to warrant this case study on its own merits. However, this book also presents some of the broader concerns of public policy. It contributes to our understanding of policy proliferation. In recent years, the government has developed a propensity to intervene in the economy. For example, federal agricultural policy has been described as "a complex web of interventions covering output markets, input markets, trade, public good investments, renewable and exhaustible natural resources, regulation of externalities, education, and marketing and distribution of food products."[9] A historical review of these public policies reveals the tension in the government's arguably contradictory actions.[10] Public policy toward tobacco also illustrates this conflicting approach.[11] Additional examples include nuclear power, the oil industry, and automobiles.[12]

Some degree of policy proliferation is inevitable in the American system. A pluralistic and democratic society tends toward incrementalism and compromise—features that encourage the proliferation of smaller interventions rather than comprehensive unilateral policies. Separation of powers at the federal level increases the likelihood of multiple sources of intervention, with each branch employing different tools and involving different constituencies. Our national government also shares power with the fifty states.[13] Thus, multiple layers of regulation have become the norm, not the exception, which is particularly true in the health care delivery and regulation system because of its complexity.

This book on medical device technology may have more general relevance to other areas of the economy. Of course, perfect generalizations cannot always be drawn from a specific case; each area has individual characteristics, and the variety of prescriptions will inevitably differ. However, the search for patterns and relationships in the evolution of various policies, and the study of private-sector responses to them, may be instructive for other areas of business-government relations. This chapter will first familiarize the reader with the patient and then establish the framework for the diagnostic process.

THE PATIENT: THE MEDICAL DEVICE INDUSTRY

Defining a Medical Device

The term *medical device* is often used synonymously with medical products, medical equipment and supplies, or medical technology. As a working definition, that of the Federal Food, Drug, and Cosmetic Act seems appropriate: a medical device is "an instrument, apparatus, implement, machine, contrivance, implant, in vitro reagent, or other similar or related article" that is intended for use in "the diagnosis of disease or other conditions [or the] cure, mitigation, treatment, or prevention of disease [or] intended to affect the structure or any function of the body of man, which does not achieve any of its principal intended purposes through chemical action within or on the body of man or other animals and which is not dependent upon being metabolized for the achievement of any of its principal purposes."[14]

The definition is less complicated than it may first appear. Basically, devices include health care items other than drugs. Devices used for diagnosis of disease include X-ray machines, scopes for viewing parts of the body, including stethoscopes and bronchoscopes, and heart monitoring equipment, to name a few. Devices used for cure or treatment include scalpels and more complicated surgical tools, lithotripsy devices that crush kidney stones with ultrasonic waves, and balloon catheters that clean out plaque formations on arteries. Examples of products that affect the structure or function of the body include artificial lenses to correct impaired vision, diaphragms or intrauterine devices used for birth control, and cardiac pacemakers to regulate heart rhythms.

The term *medical devices* can be distinguished from *medical products,* which includes both drugs and medical devices despite the distinct biomedical properties of each. Medical devices do include, but are not limited to, all nonpharmaceutical medical equipment and supplies. The term *medical technology* is even broader; the Office of Technology Assessment (OTA) has defined medical technology as "drugs, devices, and medical and surgical procedures used in medical care, and the organizational and supportive systems within which such care is provided."[15] Thus, devices are only one part of medical technology.

Medical devices include thousands of products currently produced by over 3,500 U.S. firms. The term encompasses all supplies and equipment used in hospitals from bedpans to sophisticated monitoring devices, diagnostic products from X-rays and lab kits to complex innovations such as magnetic resonance imaging and ultrasound, and nonpharmaceutical treatment products from bandages to laser surgery equipment. Outside the hospital, medical devices are found in physicians' offices, from stethoscopes and blood pressure cuffs to automated desktop blood analyzers and portable electrocardiograph (EKG) machines. Medical devices are also used in the home, including over-the-counter articles such as pregnancy test kits and heating pads.

Use of the definition crafted by the Food and Drug Administration (FDA) is noteworthy. First, in that this book explores the complex interrelationship between the government and the producers of devices, it is interesting that it was the FDA, a government agency, that first struggled with a precise definition of medical devices in order to formulate regulatory policy. Indeed, government helped to shape the industry by defining who was in or out for regulatory purposes. It is also interesting to note that the definition is residual, defining medical devices as products that are essentially nondrugs—reflecting the fact that the FDA regulated drugs long before medical devices were considered an important part of health care.[16] As the number and complexity of these nondrugs grew, a residual, catch-all category had to be carved out. This history explains why federal regulation treats the device category as a stepchild to the more clearly identifiable drug category.

Inevitably, as in most definitions, there remain some gray areas. For example, the swimming pool that one may use to alleviate back pain generally would not be considered a device, at least for regulatory purposes. Sometimes confusion arises between the treatment process and the product because in many cases the treatment cannot be given without a particular medical device. For example, a patient cannot receive electroshock treatment without an electroshock device. Thus, some efforts to regulate the device were thinly disguised attempts to ban the treatment.

Unfortunately, the FDA definition, which works well enough for regulatory purposes, is different from the categories traditionally used by government to collect data on the industry that produces medical devices. The Census of Manufactures contains comprehensive industry statistics compiled by the U.S. Department of Commerce, Bureau of the Census. These data group medical products into five Standard Industrial Classifications (SIC codes), including designations for surgical and medical instruments, surgical appliances and supplies, X-ray, electromedical, and electrotherapeutic apparatus, dental equipment, and ophthalmic goods (see table 1). The data in these classifications capture an estimated 50 to 75 percent of products defined as medical devices by the FDA.[17] In the aggregate, these data, while imperfect, are sufficient to evaluate trends in the industry.

Distinguishing Medical Products from Other Consumer Goods

Health care, like education, has never been officially considered a fundamental right under the U.S. Constitution. However, many of our health policies reflect the view that health care, like education, is a form of entitlement, a human right, rather than a privilege for the few. Social welfare programs have been designed to ensure that the elderly, the disabled, and the poor receive adequate, or at least minimal, health care services.

Table 1. Primary SIC Codes for Medical Devices

SIC code[a]	Product class	Product examples
3693	X-ray, electromedical, and electrotherapeutic apparatus	Irradiation equipment Pacemakers Ultrasonic scanners Dializers
3841	Surgical and medical supplies	Bone drills Catheters Hospital furniture
3842	Surgical appliances and supplies	Surgical dressings Crutches Sutures
3843	Dental equipment and supplies	Sterilizers Drills Teeth
3851	Ophthalmic goods	Eyeglass lenses Contact lenses Eyeglass frames

Sources: Department of Commerce, Bureau of the Census, *1982 Census of Manufactures,* Industry Series 36F, 38B (Washington, D.C., 1985). Reprinted from Susan Bartlett Foote, "From Crutches to CT Scans: Business-Government Relations and Medical Product Innovation, "*Research in Corporate Social Performance and Policy* 8 (1986):3–28.

[a]"SIC" is an abbreviation for "Standard Industrial Code."

Clearly, medical products, including both drugs and devices, are deeply embedded in and inextricably linked to health care.

The social benefits associated with medical products distinguish them from other consumer goods. Economists use the term *merit goods* to describe products that have greater significance to society than other consumer goods.[18] Unlike toasters, lawnmowers, or home computers, medical products, and their availability and affordability, raise humanitarian as well as economic issues. As a result, tension has existed between the economics of medical care and the social side of health. For example, at the turn of the century, entrepreneurial scientists took out patents and channeled the profits into further research, their supporting institutions, or their own pockets. However, traditional medical ethics made this practice questionable for health innovations. "Medicine was ensnared, as usual, in complications resulting from its peculiar combination of business and social service."[19]

We have not resolved this "peculiar" combination today. A recent article on financial issues for end-stage renal disease (ESRD) patients asks: "[I]s it a good idea to motivate patients . . . to choose their kidney dialysis units on the basis of price as well as medical quality, personal convenience, and other important factors?"[20] It is difficult to imagine advising consumers of automobiles or financial services to ignore price solely in the interests of quality or convenience. In essence, important and long-standing social values undergird our views of health care and are reflected in the public policies that have emerged.

Distinguishing Medical Devices from Drugs

Although pharmaceuticals provide the closest analogy to medical devices, we should not assume that drug and device issues are identical. Both drugs and devices are essential for the treatment and diagnosis of disease, but there are very important differences as well. Recalling the FDA definition, we know that drugs and devices operate through different biomedical mechanisms—most drugs are metabolized, and devices are not. The size and the composition of the marketplace and the range of producers differ in the two industries.

Of course, drugs and medical devices are often used in concert; for example, syringes and intravenous equipment deliver drugs directly into the body. Innovative skin patches allow gradual absorption of chemicals through the skin for various medical treatments, such as for motion sickness. Drugs and devices may offer alternative treatments. Patients may choose chemotherapy, a drug treatment, over surgery, a procedure, to eradicate cancer; women can choose among birth control pills (drugs), diaphragms, and IUDs (devices) to prevent pregnancy.

The governmental distinction between drugs and medical devices is more than a biomedical nicety. Device technologies range from lasers to computer systems to implanted materials. Because of that diversity, the nature of the medical equipment and the costs associated with its purchase and use vary much more widely than for drugs. That is not to say that all pharmaceuticals are cheap. Indeed, recent introductions, particularly products based on biotechnology, carry high price tags. Tissue plasminogen activator (TPA), a drug for treatment of stroke victims, can cost as much as $5,000 a dose.[21] Recent controversies over the high price of zidovudine (AZT), one of the few effective drugs for AIDS patients, raises the same issue. However, price variability in devices is still much broader. Devices range from simple products, such as crutches and bandages, to high-cost capital equipment, such as laboratory blood analyzers, lithotripsy equipment, and magnetic resonance imaging machines that cost several million dollars. Unlike drugs, such equipment may require maintenance, specially designed facilities, and specially trained operators and are subject to depreciation and deterioration. Other devices, such as components for kidney dialysis, raise important questions of reuse not relevant for drugs.

In addition, the medical devices market may differ from the drug market. While hospital pharmacies generate sales, physicians generally order prescription drugs for individual patients, and consumers can purchase over-the-counter (OTC) drugs directly. The primary purchasers of medical equipment are hospitals, which rank ahead of physicians, ambulatory care centers, and individuals. Hospital purchasing patterns are extremely sensitive to changing reimbursement policies by third-party payers.

There are significant distinctions between drugs and devices on the supply side as well. Because of the range of technologies embedded in medical device production, a widely diverse group of firms consider themselves part of the medical device industry. In pharmaceuticals, the top one hundred companies market 90 percent of the drugs.[22] The device industry is not nearly as concentrated: currently, over 3,500 device companies produce several thousand products. These companies range from those also known for drugs, such as Johnson & Johnson and Pfizer, to electronic giants, such as General Electric and Hewlett-Packard. In addition, there are many smaller companies concentrating exclusively on medical devices, such as Alza Corporation, which specializes in innovative drug delivery systems, and Medtronic, the leader in heart pacemakers and heart valves. Others have diversified. For example, SpaceLabs, now owned by Bristol-Myers/Squibb, applied technologies that were developed for the space program to produce a variety of monitoring and data-recording devices.

With all this diversity, it helps to consider medical device producers as a single industry. While this industry is many industries, in one sense, because no substitutability exists among all products, there is a commonality of buyers—hospitals, clinics, laboratories, physicians, and patients. However, there is a commonality in use in a broad sense—the products affect the function of the body and/or treat disease. Finally, it is the peculiar set of government health policies that have shaped the performance of this industry. All companies are, to some extent, offspring of the same set of policies, and this brings us full circle to the FDA definition of medical devices. The industry is unified by its relationship to government, both because it is defined by government and because of its symbiotic relationship to it.

THE PROCESS: A DIAGNOSTIC FRAMEWORK

As this study explores the interaction between innovative medical devices and government, an understanding of both innovation and public policy is required.

Innovation Defined

Put most simply, innovation has been defined as certain technical knowledge about how to do things better than the existing state of the art.[23] Innovation can be seen broadly as a process leading to technical change, or the concept can be more narrowly applied to a specific new product or technique.

The value of innovation to sustain economic growth and competitiveness and to improve the quality of life is not in question. Yet a clear understanding of how and why innovation occurs remains elusive. There is extensive literature, primarily in economics, on ways to model innovation.[24] Despite these continuing efforts, however, other scholars of innovation have concluded that the forces that make for innovation are so numerous and intricate that they are not fully understood.[25]

It is generally agreed, however, that certain stages are essential to the innovative process. Figure 2 illustrates the relevant stages.

The innovative process begins with *science,* which involves the systematic study of phenomena purely to add to the sum total of human knowledge.[26] Drawing on a science base, technology is directed toward use and has two phases: invention and development. Invention is the first confidence that something should work and involves testing to demonstrate that it does work. Development encompasses a wide range of activities by which technical methods are applied to the new invention so that the task is more precisely defined, the search more specific, and the chances of success more susceptible to measure. In John Jewkes's words, "Invention is the stage at which the scent is first picked up, development the stage at which the hunt is in full cry."[27]

Finally, at the end of the development stage, technical considerations give way to market concerns. Experts have broken this stage into adoption and diffusion. Once a product has been adopted by the relevant decision makers, diffusion rates depend on a variety of market factors.

For purposes of simplicity, this book distills the stages into two main categories. Science, invention, and development lead to the creation of the product itself—described here as *discovery.* The second stage—decisions to adopt and use a product—is captured by the term *distribution.*

While simplification is helpful for discussion, it is important not to forget the complexity of the process. The existence of one element in the innovation stream does not ensure forward movement. Scientific understanding does not always produce applied technical development. However, the converse appears to be true: the sequence of innovation cannot occur without all elements. There can be no invention without science. For example, despite commitment to find a cure for cancer or AIDS, the necessary products await greater scientific understanding of the diseases. Moreover, the process is not perfectly linear. For many innovations, early prototypes are tried by physicians, who may

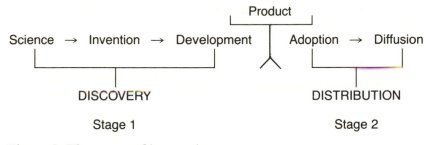

Figure 2. The stages of innovation.

encourage inventors to modify the product. Indeed, device innovation often is an iterative process involving inventors, physicians, and, occasionally, patients as well.

This innovative process can be illustrated by example. Infant mortality resulting from premature birth is a serious medical problem. Assume that physicians observed that pure oxygen is beneficial, but excessive oxygen may lead to blindness or death in the premature infant. The discovery stage would require knowledge of human physiology and of the role of oxygen. At the invention stage, the innovator would design a prototype for a mechanism to deliver the oxygen in appropriate amounts. That would require engineering expertise, such as a meter to measure oxygen flow and so on. The development stage would involve the production of the product.

Once the product is designed and constructed, the distribution stage becomes relevant. The inventor has to persuade physicians and/or hospitals to adopt the new invention, and diffusion measures how many products had been purchased to treat premature infants. Clearly, important factors arise that help or hinder the progress of the oxygen device along the innovation continuum. Questions of funding (who supports the inventor?), natural resources (is there an adequate supply of oxygen for the products?), and costs (can hospitals afford to buy the invention?) arise.

We can understand much of the medical device industry in relation to the traditional model of innovation. The industry is a business, subject to many of the same economic forces that confront all highly innovative industries. We need to know how technology is transferred, how firms are organized to facilitate competitiveness, what economic strategies work, and so forth. However, in the medical device industry, as in many other areas of the economy, government policy has intervened at virtually every stage of the innovative process. Thus, to understand innovation, we must understand something of the public policy process as well.

Public Policy

Policymaking is the process of setting goals for the public good and implementing strategies to attain them. Every public policy is the outcome of an institutional decision. Public institutions, such as regulatory agencies or state courts, are themselves creatures of the political process. They have characteristics derived from their unique history and organization. In response to political, administrative, or legal pressures, public institutions can change. To understand public policy, then, we must be well grounded in the literature on bureaucracies, the judiciary, and the legislative process.[28]

The public policies that affect medical device innovation must be understood in institutional, political, and legal contexts. History helps to establish the political and social context in which the policy intervention was introduced. For medical devices specifically, the institutions that set public policy include the National Institutes of Health (NIH), the FDA, the Medicare and Medicaid bureaucracies (the Health Care Financing Administration at the federal level for Medicare and many various departments of health in each state for Medicaid administration), the state and federal courts, and a variety of other assessment and regulatory entities.

Each policy must also be understood in terms of the social values that motivated the initial intervention. Like the concept of innovation, the concept of *value* is elusive. The term has been given so many meanings by economists, philosophers, and the public that no precise definition emerges.[29] For the purposes of our discussion, however, *value* is used to reflect social preferences—preferences communicated by the public or interest groups to decision makers for implementation through the public policy process.

For example, the public values product safety. The public policy that manifests safety is government regulation of certain products, including medical devices. How well that value is carried out depends upon the institutional commitment to it (the politics of the FDA), the structure and the jurisdiction of the institution (what the law empowers FDA to do and not do), and the response of the regulated industry. As we begin to think about reform and change, it is imperative not to lose sight of the underlying values the original policies represent. The relevant questions include: Can we achieve those values more efficiently in other ways? Are the values outdated or superseded by newer ones?

Again, for clarity, we must begin to simplify the complicated policy environment. Because we are interested in the impact of these policies on innovation, we can categorize them in relation to that process. Public policies, regardless of source or structure, tend either to promote innovation by accelerating the progress of a new product along the innovation stream or to inhibit the flow of innovation through barriers along the route.

The Matrix

The development of a matrix helps to illustrate the interrelationship between public policy and innovation. In figure 3, the stages of the innovation continuum (from discovery to distribution) are on the horizontal axis. The two identified types of public policy (promote or inhibit) appear on the vertical axis.

Each box in the matrix contains examples of policies that reflect the coordinates. Thus, policies in box 1 promote innovation at the stage of discovery, and policies in box 4 inhibit innovation at the distribution stage. The matrix provides the organizing framework for the discussion in subsequent chapters.

Chapter 2 chronicles the evolution of innovation in the private sector and the preconditions for subsequent policy interventions. In the first half of this century, medical device technology and government institutions were quite independent and engaged in little meaningful interaction. Yet there were signs of change. Technological development was taking place in the private sector, and inventors overcame significant barriers to pro-

	Discovery	Distribution
Promote	1. National Institutes of Health (NIH) Space & Defense Spinoffs	2. Hill-Burton Hospital Construction Funds Medicare/Medicaid
Inhibit	3. Regulation (FDA) Product Liability	4. Certificate of Need Cost Containment Technology Assessment

Figure 3. The policy matrix.

duce a variety of innovations. Public attitudes about the government's role in the innovative process underwent important and perceptible shifts, and public institutions were established that later would play pivotal roles in the device industry. Interaction came later. In terms of both technology development and government policy, World War II provided the transition to the modern environment.

Part II (chapters 3 through 8) follows the chronology of the boxes in the matrix. Policy trends are easily identified, as the numbers reflect the last four decades. In general, the policies of the 1950s (box 1) were dominated by promotion of innovation at the discovery stage, and the 1960s (box 2) saw promotion at the distribution stage, with consequent benefits for both discovery and distribution. The 1970s and 1980s did not completely reverse these trends, in that the policies initiated earlier continued. However, new concerns led to efforts to inhibit innovation. In the 1970s (box 3), significant efforts to increase regulation inhibited discovery; in the 1980s (box 4), concern about cost containment led to policies to inhibit product distribution. The chronology is not exact because some of the regulatory antecedents appeared before the policies were enforced. (The FDA had authority to regulate medical devices as early as 1938; the extension of authority with regulatory teeth, however, came in 1976.)

Subsequent policies did not replace earlier ones. Rather, policies were layered one on top of the other, so that public policy affected innovation at every step. To help us understand the proliferation of policies, each intervention is discussed in relation to the politics of its creation and evolution, the interest groups involved, the goals of the policymakers, and the changes over time.

Each chapter in part II relates to a box in the matrix presented in figure 3. Chapter 3 addresses how government policy promotes discovery (box 1). The NIH is the primary federal organization charged with supporting biomedical research, which has been accomplished through grants to researchers, primarily in universities. Some recent initiatives, most notably the Artificial Heart Program (AHP) at NIH, which is modeled on the experiences of the space program, have targeted specific device technologies. Additionally, chapter 3 looks at government sponsored research in space and defense that has had some interesting effects on medical device technology. Also discussed are recent political efforts to realign the key research institutions—universities, government scientists, and the industry—so that medical technology is transferred from the basic science of the laboratory into the hands of product producers. The chapter evaluates these three initiatives in relation to the medical device industry.

Chapter 4 focuses on policies that promote distribution (box 2). Public policy has played a pivotal role in shaping the size and the composition of the medical device market. Federal and state governments have developed a complex set of policies to pay for health care services. After years of disinterest in health services, federal spending on the growth of the hospital infrastructure began after World War II. Chapter 4 describes how the public role expanded significantly with the enactment of Medicare and Medicaid in the 1960s. The primary health policy goal undergirding public payment is to increase access to health care for those previously excluded, including the elderly, the disabled, and the indigent. Although these programs did not directly address the medical device industry, their impact on that industry was dramatic. Government programs continue to inject billions of dollars into the medical marketplace every year, and medical technologies are a primary beneficiary. The design of these payment policies dramatically and idiosyncratically affects the size of the market for particular medical technologies.

A few examples illustrate the point. According to some estimates, in 1982 the government paid for over 41 percent of all medical expenditures.[30] The payment structure favored hospital based technologies over nonhospital products. Intensive care units, full of new life-support and monitoring equipment, were virtually unknown in 1960; in 1984, they accounted for 8 percent of all hospital beds. Congress extended Medicare coverage for all end-stage renal disease (ESRD) patients in 1972. Kidney dialysis, virtually nonexistent in 1960, was used by 80,000 patients in 1984 at a cost to the government of $1.8 billion.[31]

The 1970s brought a new set of concerns to the policy arena— primarily product safety. Chapter 5 explores how the government inhibited discovery of medical devices through safety regulations (box 3). Regulation of medical devices is the primary vehicle for reducing risks of adverse reactions to these products. The federal government and, to a lesser extent, the states have recognized that certain medical products present unacceptable risks and require government intervention through safety and efficacy regulation.

Food and drug regulation dates back to the turn of the century. Congress extended the jurisdiction of the FDA to cover medical devices in 1938; the FDA acquired significantly more extensive regulatory powers under the 1976 Medical Device Amendments to the Federal Food, Drug, and Cosmetic Act, one of the many pieces of consumer protection legislation of the 1970s. The stated goal of these amendments was to "provide for the *safety and effectiveness* of medical devices intended for human use."[32] The FDA's jurisdiction is over producers, and its regulations affect firms at the development stage. Cardiac pacemakers and intrauterine devices (IUDs) are used in this chapter to illustrate the impact of regulation on device technology. Because the law focuses on perceived risks associated with medical devices, the riskier the product, the more likely it will encounter the inhibiting forces of the FDA.

Chapter 6 continues the discussion of policies that inhibit device discovery (box 3). Although it has antecedents in early common-law rules, there was an explosion in product liability suits in the 1970s. Product liability seeks to inhibit the manufacture and use of devices if they are determined to be unsafe. However, state courts use completely different tools from FDA regulators to accomplish this substantially similar goal. Liability law in general has a less well-recognized, but clearly related, health mission. Its goal is to compensate individuals injured by defective products and to deter others from producing harmful products. It functions as a part of the health care system in that income to pay for medical costs, as well as noneconomic damage, is transferred from the producers of products to the consumers of products. It is essentially a form of insurance coverage for risk. The law includes both a compensatory and a safety function. The product liability system applies to all consumer products; medical products are included in this broad net. Product liability law, in terms of both the costs and availability of insurance and the consequences of lawsuits, can have a significant, indeed a crippling, impact on some producers.

Chapter 7 analyzes the series of recently imposed mechanisms that inhibit distribution of medical devices (box 4). These policies focus on cost containment rather than on safety, though some seek to control costs through evaluation of product quality. Concern about health care costs in the 1970s and 1980s has affected the momentum of federal and state payment programs. Efforts to restructure the system to control costs have had substantial effects on some segments of the medical device marketplace. Cost-containment strategies began with state based Certificate of Need programs and expanded to a variety of cost-control forms through technology assessment mechanisms. The goal of assessment processes is to ensure that only the "best" technologies are distributed—other technologies should be abandoned. Chapter 7 focuses on federal efforts to institutionalize technology assessment beyond the existing policymaking bodies. In addition, the new payment system under Medicare, known as the Prospective Payment System (PPS), was instituted to control the wildly escalating costs of Medicare. This program has created a new set of idiosyncratic effects on medical device technology.

Chapter 8 introduces the emerging issues of a global marketplace. These issues do not appear within the matrix because it is

| POLICIES TO | R&D Funds | | Payment Policies | |
| PROMOTE | ------------------> | | ---------------------> | |

| | ∿∿∿∿ | Discovery | ∿∿∿∿ | Distribution | ∿∿∿∿ |

POLICIES TO	<------------------	<---------------------	<-----------------------
INHIBIT	Safety	Product Liability	Cost Controls
	Regulation		Diffusion Controls

Figure 4. Policies affecting medical device innovation.

unclear whether the international market and the policies of foreign governments regarding medical technology will help domestic medical device producers (that is, promote distribution) or pose a competitive threat to domestic producers (that is, inhibit distribution). Through a brief look at three major markets—Japan, the emerging European Community, and China—these challenges will be assessed.

Part III provides a prognosis. Returning to the innovation continuum, the discussion in chapter 9 falls into three sections (figure 4). The first analyzes the present policy environment at both the discovery and the distribution stages, with illustrations of creative industry strategies that respond to policy incentives. The second section discusses pending policy reforms and their possible effect on the flow of new products. The third section discusses interactions among the various policies that are the inevitable consequences of policy proliferation. Some ways to improve the policy process are discussed.

Chapter 10 looks to the future. The contributions of medical devices to the fight against disease have been critical. However, there are dangers posed by misuse and overuse. The medical arms race must be managed with an understanding of the economic, political, and moral dimensions of medical technology.

The development and application of an analytical framework to the medical device industry only scratches the surface. Further empirical work is necessary to improve our understanding of medical technologies, of the process of innovation, and of the impact of government institutions on the private sector. It is hoped that the issues raised in this book will encourage this research. We must strive for rational policy reform grounded in an understanding of the values and goals of our health care system.

Finally, this study makes clear that policy proliferation is inherent in our political system and reflects the complexity of technology. The system has many benefits, but it also has costs and limitations. It is useful to step back and view the whole landscape to observe the dynamic interactions between the public and the private sectors. In the case of our patient—medical devices—reform may indeed be a matter of life and death.

2

PRECONDITIONS FOR INTERACTION

> When my grandfather George had a stroke he
> was led into the house and put to bed, and the
> Red Men sent lodge brothers to sit with him to
> exercise the curative power of brotherhood. . . .
> Ida Rebecca called upon modern technology to
> help George. From a mail-order house she or-
> dered a battery-operated galvanic device which
> applied the stimulation of low-voltage electrical
> current to his paralyzed limbs. . . . In Morrison-
> ville death was a common part of life. It came for
> the young as relentlessly as it came for the old. To
> die antiseptically in a hospital was almost un-
> known. In Morrisonville death still made house
> calls.
>
> Russell Baker
> *Growing Up*

Journalist Russell Baker's description of his grandfather's death
is typical of American health care in the 1920s.[1] The technological changes that characterized agricultural and industrial
production had not yet come to medicine.[2] Physicians had limited knowledge, and commonly prescribed therapies were improved diets, more exercise, and cleaner environments, not the
highly technological interventions customary today.[3] Doctors
held out little hope for treatment of most illnesses; consumers
like Baker's grandmother often turned to folk remedies or miracle cures. Hospitals were shunned as places where destitute
people without family went to die.[4] Government played a negli-
gible role in health care, and any costs of treatment would have

been borne by the Baker family, or the treatment foregone if money were not available.

During the first four decades of the twentieth century, innovation in health sciences did occur. Important breakthroughs included improved aseptic surgery techniques, sulfa drugs, and vaccines to treat, and prevent the spread of, infectious diseases. The nascent medical device industry assisted in the advancement of medical science. There were increasingly sophisticated scopes for observation of internal bodily functions and advances in the laboratory equipment that permitted precise measurement of biochemical phenomena. However, quack devices proliferated in addition to legitimate innovations. Many fraudulent devices promising miracle cures capitalized on new discoveries in the fields of electricity and magnetism. The galvanic device purchased to treat Baker's grandfather was typical of popular quack products of the time. Unfortunately for the industry as a whole, these quack devices contributed to the public perception that medical devices were marginal to advanced medical care.

This chapter illustrates how individuals and firms overcame structural and scientific barriers to innovation in the private sector. Various private individuals and corporations managed to bridge these gaps. As a result, the medical device sector enjoyed modest and steady growth.

What is most interesting to the modern reader is the limited role that government played in medical technology innovation. However, seeds of the subsequent multiple roles of government were sown in this early period. By the eve of World War II, several public institutions had been created that would later significantly affect device development. The National Institutes of Health (NIH) would promote medical discovery; the Food and Drug Administration (FDA) would inhibit it. Government involvement in medical device distribution, however, did not occur until somewhat later. World War II accelerated the process of device innovation because of government involvement in the war effort; it both created a demand for medical innovations and overcame the public's reluctance to accept a government role in health policy.

The foundation for subsequent business-government interac-

tion in medical device innovation had been laid. To use our
analogy, the preconditions for later prescriptions to treat our
patient were set; full-blown medical intervention awaited the
1950s.

TAKING THE PATIENT'S HISTORY:
INDUSTRY OVERVIEW, 1900–1940
Barriers to Device Innovation in the Private Sector

Throughout the eighteenth and nineteenth centuries there was
no continuous scientific tradition in America. Medical science
depended upon foreign discoveries, which were dominated by
Britain in the early nineteenth century, France at midcentury,
and Germany in the last half of the century. The lack of research
has been attributed to the dearth of certain conditions and facilities essential to medical studies.[5] The absence of dynamic basic
science obviously limited the possibility of technological breakthroughs.

However, the early part of the twentieth century witnessed a
rise in private sector commitment to basic medical science. Phil-
anthropists, intrigued by possibilities of improvements in health
sciences, began to endow private research facilities. The first was
the Rockefeller Institute, founded in New York City in 1902. A
number of other philanthropic foundations were established in
the Rockefeller's wake, including the Hooper Institute for Medical Research, the Phipps Institute in Philadelphia, and the Cush-
ing Institute in Cleveland. This period has been called the "Era
of Private Support."[6] These efforts improved the scientific research base in America, but it was still weak.

Compounding this weakness were barriers between basic science and medical practice. During the nineteenth century, prac-
ticing physicians had little concern for, or interest in, medical
research. Most doctors practiced traditional medicine, relying
on their small arsenal of tried-and-true remedies. However, in
the first decades of the twentieth century, medicine began to
change profoundly, which led to organizational permutations
through which the medical profession became more scientific

and rigorous.[7] University medical schools began to grow as the need for integration of medical studies and basic sciences was acknowledged. Support for medical schools tied research to practice and rewarded doctors for research based medical education. By the end of this period, then, many of the problems associated with lack of basic medical science research had begun to be addressed. However, by modern standards, the commitment to research was extremely small.

As our discussion of innovation revealed, basic scientific research must be linked to invention and development. In other words, there must be mechanisms by which technology is transferred from one stage in the innovation continuum to another. In the nineteenth century, there were serious gaps between basic medical science and applied engineering, which is an essential part of medical device development. American engineering education rarely involved research.[8] Engineers were trained in technical schools but had few university contacts thereafter. Furthermore, manufacturers had little patience for the ivory towers of university science; they looked instead for profits in the marketplace. Engineering practitioners emphasized applying knowledge to the design of technical systems. Thus, engineers based in private companies were cautious about the developments of advanced technology, preferring to make gradual moves in known directions.[9] Producers were slow to take advantage of any advances in research in the United States or abroad. Established industries tended to ignore science and to depend on empirical inventions for new developments.[10] Patents for medical products did accelerate at the turn of the century, but a majority of them represented engineering shortcuts, not true innovations.[11]

A few very large corporations addressed this problem through the creation of in-house research laboratories that combined basic science and applied engineering. These institutions focused primarily on incremental product development, but innovative technologies did appear. Thus, while the gap between universities and corporations did not close, some firms became research-oriented through the establishment of independent laboratories. Companies with large laboratories included American

Telephone and Telegraph and General Electric (GE). One major medical device, the X-ray, emerged from GE's research lab. It will be described at greater length shortly.

Further barriers to product development arose from the uneasy relationship between product manufacturers and both university researchers and medical practitioners. A rash of patents were applied for following the development of aseptic surgery. Between 1880 and 1890, the Patent Office granted about 1,200 device patents. The debate that raged over patents of medical products illustrates the tension between health care and profits. Universities generally resisted patenting innovations for several reasons. They valued the free flow of scientific knowledge among scholars. They faced hard questions raised about how to allocate profits of the final result because of the interconnectedness of basic scientific research. They were also concerned that a profit orientation within academia would discourage the practice of sharing scientific knowledge for the betterment of all.[12]

Innovations produced by medical inventors raised additional ethical problems. Often the physician-inventors stood by while commercial organizations exploited remedies based on their work. The medical profession had a traditional ethic against profiting from patents, and the debates about the ethics of patenting medical products continued through this period.[13] For example, the Jefferson County Medical Society of Kentucky stated that it "condemns as unethical the patenting of drugs or medical appliances for profit whether the patent be held by a physician or be transferred by him to some university or research fund, since the result is the same, namely, the deprivation of the needy sick of the benefits of many new medical discoveries through the acts of medical men."[14]

Dr. Chevalier Jackson, a noted expert in diseases of the throat, developed many instruments to improve diagnostic and surgical techniques. In his autobiography in 1938, he wrote:

> When I became interested in esophagoscopy, direct laryngoscopy, and a little later in bronchoscopy, the metal-working shop at home became a busy place. In it were worked out most of the mechanical problems of foreign body endoscopy. Sometimes the finished instrument was made. At other times only the models were made to demonstrate to the instrument maker the problem and the method

of solution. This had the advantage that the instrument was ever afterward available to all physicians. No instrument that I devised was ever patented. It galled me in early days, when I devised my first bronchoscope, to find that a similar lamp arrangement had been patented by a mechanic for use on a urethroscope, and the mechanic insisted that the use of such an arrangement on a bronchoscope was covered. Caring nothing for humanity, the patentee threatened a lawsuit unless his patent right was recognized during the few remaining years it had left to run.[15]

Not all physicians and scientists shared these views, but there was clearly a conflict between the perception of medical technology for the public good and the pursuit of profits, one that created a possible barrier to a full exploitation of the marketplace.

The last barrier to innovation in the medical field was the absence of a sizable market for the available products. In 1940, on the eve of World War II, total spending on health care in the United States amounted to $3.987 billion, or $29.62 per person per year. Health care spending accounted for only 4 percent of GNP. Patients paid directly for about 85 percent of costs. A small number of people received public assistance in city or county hospitals; there was virtually no private insurance coverage.[16] There was no buffer for individuals and families in hard times, and health care was often sacrificed when family income was limited.

The market for medical technology remained small by modern standards. The number of hospital beds was low in comparison to present population-to-bed ratios. Doctors' offices had little technological equipment. Fortunately, the small market did not deter researchers in some cases. For example, a 1914 study by engineers at General Electric concluded that new X-ray tubes would be more expensive than earlier ones and that the market would be too small to justify manufacture. Nonetheless, the management insisted that production proceed, noting that "the tube should be exploited in such a way as to confer a public benefit, feeling that it is a device which is useful to humanity and that we cannot afford to take an arbitrary or even perhaps any ordinary commercial position with regard to it."[17]

Because of this altruistic view, General Electric soon dominated the X-ray market and later turned a tidy profit on the enterprise. Obviously, however, most producers and inventors could not afford to ignore "ordinary commercial" considerations.

Bridging the Gaps

Innovation did occur despite the severe limitations in the private sector. Several examples of device innovation illustrate how these limitations were overcome.

Individual Initiative

One way to overcome institutional barriers to technology transfer was for an individual to fulfill several essential roles. Arnold Beckman, the founder of Beckman Instruments, was a scientist, engineer, and entrepreneur and thus had expertise in all the necessary stages of innovation.[18] As an assistant professor of chemistry at the California Institute of Technology in the early 1930s, he was called upon to solve technical problems that involved chemistry and then engaged in entrepreneurial activities with the results. His first business venture was to create a special ink formula that would not clog the inking mechanism in a postal meter. Because existing companies would not make the special formula, Beckman founded the National Inking Appliance Company in 1934.

Beckman soon undertook additional projects with applications for science and medicine. At the request of agricultural interests, he invented a meter to measure the acidity of lemon juice that had been heavily dosed with sulfur dioxide. Using electronic skills he had developed at Bell Labs as a graduate student, Beckman designed the first acidimeter to measure the acidity or alkalinity of any solution containing water. He formed Beckman Instruments in 1935 to produce these acidimeters and discovered a market among some of his former professors at a meeting of the American Chemical Society.

In recalling the founding of his company, Beckman noted, "We were lucky because we came into the market at just the time that acidity was getting to be recognized as a very important variable to be controlled, whether it be in body chemistry or food production."[19] In 1939 he quit teaching to run the business fulltime. Beckman's substantial contribution to the war effort, and the benefits the firm reaped as a consequence, will be discussed in a subsequent section. His company later became one of the major medical technology firms in America.[20] Beckman's career illustrates how a multifaceted individual, with scientific, technical, and marketing skills, could successfully produce scientific instruments despite the significant barriers to innovation in the early twentieth century.

Industrial Research Laboratories

Industrial research laboratories also served as bridges between science and technology and the market. Generally set apart from production facilities, these laboratories were staffed by people trained in science and advanced engineering and who were working toward an understanding of corporate related science and technology.[21] By setting up labs, large firms could conduct scientific research internally and profit from the discoveries. These laboratories were possible only after the period of consolidations and mergers in the late 1890s and early 1900s that led to the growth of industrial giants that had sufficient resources to fund them. Research was vital, and product development formed a large part of their competitive strategy. These large firms were well aware of scientific developments in Europe, particularly in the fields of electrochemistry, X-rays, and radioactivity, and they knew they had to stay abreast of technological change.[22]

General Electric Company, founded in 1892, created a research laboratory that was firmly established within the company by 1910. William Coolidge led research efforts on the X-ray tube, which had been discovered in Germany in the 1890s. It was widely known that X-rays had medical value in that they allowed doctors to observe bone and tissue structure without surgery. Two-element, partially evacuated tubes generated the X-rays. As they operated, the tubes produced more gas, changing the pressure and making them erratic. Coolidge substituted tungsten for platinum. It could be heated to a greater temperature without melting, while emitting less gas than platinum to achieve higher-powered and longer-lived tubes.

By 1913, the laboratory was manufacturing Coolidge's X-ray tubes on a small scale, selling 300 that year and 6,500 in 1914.[23] When the government began to place large orders of tubes for portable X-ray units for military hospitals during World War I, GE began to make significant profits. After the war, GE's management decided that the company would become a full-line X-ray supplier. GE bought the Victor X-ray company, switched its production of Coolidge tubes to Victor, and soon held a dominant position in the new and increasingly profitable medical equipment supply business.[24]

Problems of Medical Quackery

Along with these exciting breakthroughs in medical technology, a very different side of the industry flourished. The popularity of fraudulent devices, and concern about the consequences of that fraud, tainted public perception of the industry. Many people associated medical devices with quack products.[25]

When medical science offers no hope of treatment or cure, people have traditionally turned to charms and fetishes for help.[26] The desperate search for cures was a major factor in the success of all forms of health fraud, including tonics, drugs, potions, and quack devices. Indeed, it is estimated that the public spent $80 million in 1906 on patent medicines of all kinds. The proliferation of quack devices helped to generate subsequent government intervention to protect the public.

Innovative developments in scientific fields, such as electromagnetism and electricity, were often applied to lend credence to these health frauds (see figure 5). At the turn of the century, Dr. Hercules Sanché developed his Electropoise machine to aid in the "spontaneous cure of disease."[27] This device, consisting of a sealed metal cylinder attached to an uninsulated flexible cord that, in turn, attached to the wrist or ankle, supplied, according to the inventor, "the needed amount of electric force to the system and by its thermal action places the body in a condition to absorb oxygen through the lungs and pores."[28] The Oxydonor was a subsequent "improvement" that added a stick of

PROF. WILSON'S
Magneto-Conservative Garments.

The following figure represents the manner in which our Magneto-Conservative Garments are worn. It can be readily understood that they are not worn next the skin, nor have they to be dipped in acids. The dangerous character of Electric Belts charged with acid and worn next the skin is too well known to be repeated here. PROF. WILSON'S system is as distinct from these dangerous Copper and Zinc Belts as is a pine knot in an Indian's wigwam to the electric light of our stores and city streets. There need not be a sick person in America (save from accidents) if our Magneto-Conservative Underwear would become a part of the wardrobe of every lady and gentleman, as also of infants and children.

CURES

NERVOUS PROSTRATION,

KIDNEY DISEASE,

LIVER DISEASE,

LUNG TROUBLES.

RHEUMATISM,

GOUT,

STIFF JOINTS,

PARALYSIS,

LOCOMOTOR ATAXIA,

WRITER'S CRAMP,

LOSS OF MEMORY,

GIDDINESS,

VARICOSE VEINS,

AND

EVERY OTHER FORM OF DISEASE.

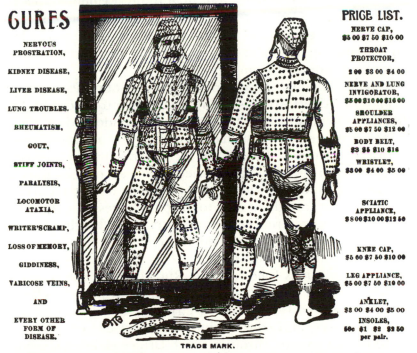

TRADE MARK.

PRICE LIST.

NERVE CAP,
$5 00 $7 50 $10 00

THROAT PROTECTOR,
2 00 $3 00 $4 00

NERVE AND LUNG INVIGORATOR,
$5 00 $10 00 $16 00

SHOULDER APPLIANCES,
$5 00 $7 50 $12 00

BODY BELT,
$3 $5 $10 $16

WRISTLET,
$3 00 $4 00 $5 00

SCIATIC APPLIANCE,
$8 00 $10 00 $12 50

KNEE CAP,
$5 00 $7 50 $10 00

LEG APPLIANCE,
$5 00 $7 50 $10 00

ANKLET,
$3 00 $4 00 $5 00

INSOLES,
50c $1 $2 $2 50
per pair.

These Garments are as puzzling to the physicians as is the wonder-working "Actina." They cure all forms of disease after the physicians fail, whether Allopath, Homœopath, Electropath or all the other Pathies of the school. These marvelous appliances will positively cure any of the following forms of disease: Prolapsus, Spinal Disease, Gout, Rheumatism, Kidney Disease, Chronic Lame Back, Paralysis, Nervous Prostration, Loss of Memory, Dyspepsia and all forms of Female Weakness or Loss of Vital Force in Man or Woman. Persons never come to us until the regular physicians have failed. Prof. Wilson practiced medicine twenty-five years, but he now seeks to make amends for having given his time to so pernicious a system "as drugging poor suffering humanity." His patented Magneto-Conservative Garments and their marvelous effects demonstrate a mind of deep research. No physician can examine the structure of these appliances and not be convinced of their value.

Send for Prof. Wilson's treatise on "Disease and its Cure," and other valuable information.

Sample of thousands of testimonials on file in our office:

A MOST REMARKABLE CURE OF DROPSY.

FLORENCE, MO.

New York & London Electric Association, Kansas City, Mo.

Gentlemen—You will excuse me for not writing to you before about my wife's case that we treated. She had the worst case of dropsy that I ever saw or heard of. It was in her system for years, and after her child was born it developed in a severe form. She was so much bloated that she could not find a chair large enough for her; in fact, I cannot describe her—she simply was awful to look at. I called in Dr. Scales; and he told me she could not last over four hours. Then I called Dr. Croferd, and he said she would be a dead woman in less than two hours. Then I called Dr. Bronson, and he shook his head and said, we will try. In the meantime I had sent for the magnetic goods. They got here on the night train. I put them on her that night and by morning had the water running out of every pore of her body, and kept doing so for three weeks, and now, after four years, I will say she has not seen a sick moment since. Her skin is soft and healthy. Your goods saved her and her child's life. Use this as you like.

Yours, with respects,

A. J. MAURY.

NEW YORK & LONDON ELECTRIC ASSOCIATION, Mfrs

929 Walnut Street,
KANSAS CITY, MO.

Figure 5. A quack device.

Source: The Bakken Archives.

carbon to the sealed, and incidentally hollow and empty, cylinder and "cured all forms of disease." The success of the Oxydonor spawned a whole cadre of imitations. There was a death knell for these "pipe and wire" therapies when the inventor of the Oxypathor was convicted of mail fraud. Evidence collected at the trial revealed that the company had sold 45,451 Oxypathors at $35 each in 1914. Considering that as late as 1940 per capita spending on health was only $29.62, the consequences of wasted expenditures seem serious.

Another fraud was based on the new field of radio communications. Dr. Albert Abrams of San Francisco introduced his "Radionics" system, which was based on the pseudomedical theory that electrons are the basic biological unit and all disease stems from a "disharmony of electronic oscillation." Dr. Abrams's diagnoses were made by placing dried blood specimens into the Radioscope. Operated with the patient facing west in a dim light, the device purported not only to diagnose illness but also to tell one's religious preference, sex, and race. At the height of its use, over 3,500 practitioners rented the device from Abrams for $200 down and $5 a month.[29]

One of Abrams's followers was Ruth Drown. She marketed the Drown Radio Therapeutic Instrument, which she claimed could prevent and cure cancer, cirrhosis, heart trouble, back pain, abscesses, and constipation. The device used a drop of blood from a patient, through which Drown claimed she could "tune in" on diseased organs and restore them to health. With two drops she could treat any patient by remote control. A larger version of her instrument was claimed to diagnose as well as to treat disease. Thousands of Californians patronized her establishment.[30]

Unfortunately for legitimate medical device producers, the prevalence of device quackery tainted the public's perception of the industry. Indeed, initial state and federal efforts to regulate the industry were in response to problems of fraud. Device fraud continues, especially for diseases like arthritis and cancer and for weight control.[31] Fraud in the industry can be seen as a market failure that subsequent government prescriptions sought to correct.

Industry Status in 1940

Despite the successes of some firms and some individuals, the medical device industry remained relatively small even as late as 1937. The Census of Manufactures, the best source of information about producers, categorized all industrial production into Standard Industrial Codes. Before 1937, the Census contained only one primary industrial category for medical products. This was SIC 3842—surgical appliances and supplies—which included items such as bandages, surgical gauze and dressings, first aid kits, and surgical and orthopedic appliances. Both the number of producers and the value of their sales in SIC 3842 were quite small until the 1930s. For example, in 1914 there were 391 establishments that shipped products valued at about $16.5 million. The number of producers rose to 445 during World War I, dropped to below 300 until the midtwenties, fell further to 250 during the depression, and reached 323 in 1937. Sales reflected the same ebb and flow, dropping from $71 million in 1929 to $51 million in 1933, and recovering to $77 million by 1937.

In the late 1920s a second classification—SIC 3843—was added for dental products and supplies. In the 1937 data, three important classifications emerged. SIC 3693 included X-ray and therapeutic apparatus. Sales of these products had occurred before this time; however, they were buried in other, nonmedical industrial categories. The industries that produced these products engaged primarily in manufacturing X-ray tubes and lamps for ultraviolet radiation. By the 1950s, the name of the code changed to X-ray, electromedical, and electrotherapeutic apparatus, reflecting the growing innovation in this field. By 1937, SIC 3693 accounted for $17 million in sales with forty-six companies producing equipment. A second new code was SIC 3841—surgical and medical instruments—which included products such as surgical knives and blades, hypodermic syringes, and diagnostic apparatus such as ophthalmoscopes. In 1937, thirty-nine companies were producing devices in this code. In that year, records began to be kept for a fifth medical product category, SIC 3851, ophthalmic goods, which included eyeglass frames, lenses, and industrial goggles and included seventy-nine companies selling about $43 million worth of goods in 1937. In all five relevant SIC codes, there were only 588 establishments with total product shipments valued at $200 million.[32]

As we have seen, there was some innovation and modest, though inconsistent, growth in the medical device industry from 1900 to 1940. New products emerged despite barriers to technology transfer at the various stages of the innovation continuum. However, innovation was frequently serendipitous, dependent on individuals and not institutionalized sufficiently to ensure a steady stream of progress. Creative entrepreneurs and industrial laboratories did play a role in overcoming obstacles for some technologies. On the other hand, the device industry was plagued with quackery and fraud.

EVOLUTION OF PUBLIC INSTITUTIONS, 1900–1940

With the exception of government procurement during World War I, the device industry grew with minimal government involvement. However, intervention was beginning during this period.

There were perceptible shifts in the public's attitude about the appropriate role of the federal government in economic and social issues. Early institutions and policies emerged that would both promote and inhibit medical innovation. How these policies evolved would influence, to a large extent, the contours of the emerging medical device industry.

Government Promotes Discovery

The general aversion toward government involvement in basic research gave way to acceptance of a public role—a change reflected in the creation of the National Institutes of Health (NIH). At the turn of the century, medical practitioners vehemently rejected any government intervention in their domain. In 1900, a well-known physician appeared before a Senate committee and declared that all the medical profession asked of Congress was no interference with its progress.[33] Even as late as 1928, Atherton Seidell, a famous chemist, stated, "We [Americans] naturally question governmental participation in scientific matters because we feel that anything having a political flavor cannot be above suspicion."[34] But, in the same year, scientist Charles Holmes Herty said, in regard to support of basic science, "I have changed my mind completely, and I feel that the Government should lead in this matter."[35]

Early government activities were primarily in the area of public health, not research. The roots of government involvement lie in the federal Hygienic Laboratory, founded in 1902 to implement the Biologics Control Act, one of the earliest pieces of U.S. health legislation. Under this act, the Hygienic Lab inspected vaccine laboratories, tested the purity of the products and issued licenses.[36] In addition, the Public Health Service was established in 1912 to address applied health issues. Neither institution had real involvement in basic sciences until World War I. On the eve of the war, the relationship between science in the private sector and science in government was in a state of equilibrium, with the private sector supporting basic research as well as some applied work and the federal government devoting its limited revenues to practical scientific work through the Hygienic Lab and the Public Health Service.[37]

The war made the government conscious of the value of science, particularly as German superiority in chemical warfare became apparent. Thus, after the war, there was more talk of public and private sector cooperation to promote science. The proposals put forward in this period, however, advocated the control and direction of research under private auspices with very limited government participation. President Coolidge did not believe in marked expansion of the governmental initiatives to promote health; he viewed medicine and science as the provinces of the private sector. In 1928, Coolidge vetoed a bill to create a National Institute of Health that would provide fellowships for research funded by private donations.[38] He stated, "I do not believe that permanency of appointment of those engaged in the professional and scientific activities of the Government is necessary for progress or accomplishment in those activities or in keeping with public policy."[39] However, the private sector was not willing to come forward single-handed with substantial funds to support this undertaking. One historian noted that this lack "was to make the concept of government funding less noxious as the years passed and the original hope dimmed."[40]

With the private sector sufficiently unresponsive, a law establishing the National Institute of Health finally passed in 1930. However, NIH expansion into a large-scale facility was nearly twenty years in the future. The NIH remained small but not totally inactive. Although Congress refused to appropriate the maximum amount during the 1930s, the NIH did receive increased monies to expand research into chronic diseases. In 1937, Congress authorized the National Cancer Institute (NCI) with legislation that sped through Congress in record time and that was unanimously supported by the Senate.[41]

However, most of the NIH's accomplishments up to World War II were responses to public health emergencies. As late as 1935, the president's Science Advisory Board concluded that no comprehensive, centrally controlled research program was desirable except for certain problems related to public health. By 1937, total federal research expenses, spread out among many federal agencies, amounted to only $124 million, and much of that was allocated to natural sciences and nonmedical technology.[42]

Despite limited funding, the NIH represented a significant change in attitude toward the role of government. During this period, the NIH research orientation was set as well. Much of its early work continued to be in the science of public health, and research support could have moved in a more applied direction. However, the NIH preferred to expand into basic research, primarily in conjunction with universities, and avoided support of applied research. In chapter 3, we shall see how the political commitment to the NIH and its research orientation affected medical device innovation.

Government Inhibits Discovery

Government promotion of medical discovery emerged alongside institutions that would later inhibit discovery. This inhibiting role for government arose in response to problems of fraud and quackery.

Fraud in food and medicine sales was nothing new, but during the 1880s and 1890s concern grew about dangerous foodstuffs in the market. Attention focused on the sale of diseased meats and milk, on adulterated food products such as a combination of inert matter, ground pepper, glucose, hayseed, and flavoring that was sold as raspberry jam. Many nostrums contained dangerous, habit-forming narcotics sold to an uninformed and unsuspecting public.[43]

States did pass laws to regulate the marketing of harmful products, but these laws were relatively ineffectual because a state could not enforce its regulations against an out-of-state manufacturer. The only recourse was to reach producers indirectly through the local retailers who handled the goods. At the federal level, Congress was not inactive; from 1879, when the House introduced the first bill designed to prevent the adulteration of food, to June 30, 1906, when the Pure Food Law was signed, 190 measures relating to problems with specific foods had been introduced.[44]

A number of important interests marshalled considerable opposition to federal intervention. States' rights Democrats from the South believed that the federal government did not have the constitutional authority to intervene in the private sector.[45] Some food producers and retailers contended that they could not sell their goods if they had to label all the ingredients. The drug industry joined the fray when a Senate bill extended the definition of drugs to include not only medicines recognized by the United States Pharmacopeia,[46] but also any substance intended for the cure, mitigation, or treatment of disease. This definition would bring the proprietary medicines within the scope of the law.[47] The Proprietary Association of America, with trade organizations of wholesale and retail druggists, immediately joined the opposition.

Commercial interests could not suppress public opinion after disclosures of adulterated foods in the muckraking press stirred up the progressive fervor. The 1905 publication of Upton Sinclair's *The Jungle*, which contained graphic images of adulterated food, including a contention that some lard was made out of the bodies of workmen who had fallen into cooking vats, provoked reform. Harvey W. Wiley, chief of the Division of Chemistry in the Department of Agriculture, became a missionary for reform. He organized the "poison squad" in 1902 and found that the volunteers who restricted their food intake to diets that included a variety of food additives, such as boric acid, benzoate of soda, and formaldehyde, suffered metabolic, digestive, and health problems.[48]

The 1906 Pure Food Act was a compromise among many diverse and competing interests. The act was very different in orientation from the subsequent drug regulation; it was intended to aid consumers in the marketplace, not to restrict access of products to the market. The act, in short, made misrepresentation illegal. A drug was deemed adulterated if it deviated from the standards of the national formularies without so admitting on the label. A drug was considered misbranded if the company sold it under a false name or in the package of another drug or if it failed to identify the presence of designated addictive substances. The authority of the federal government was limited to seizure of the adulterated or misbranded articles and prosecution of the manufacturer.[49]

It is important to remember that this was not an effort by the federal government to intervene in medical care decisions. Because there were few effective drugs in 1906 and most were purchased by consumers without the aid of physicians, drug regulation was seen as a part of food regulation, not of health care per se. Inclusion of medical devices—products used for health care but not consumed as food or drugs—does not appear to have been considered during the decades in which Congress debated food and drug legislation.

Nevertheless, the 1906 law initiated the subsequent growth of a federal role in consumer protection. The Department of Agriculture's Division of Chemistry administered the law. It was renamed the Bureau of Chemistry in 1901; its appropriation rose by a factor of five, and the number of employees grew from 110 in 1906 to 425 in 1908.[50] The Agriculture Appropriations Act of 1931 established the Food and Drug Administration (FDA) within the department.[51] It had a budget of $1.6 million and over 500 employees at the time of its name change.

Although medical devices were overlooked from 1906 to 1931, several important steps had been taken. First, there was acceptance of the federal government's role in protecting the public from adulterated and misbranded products. There was also a federal institution in place, the FDA, with expertise in regulation. As problems arose subsequently in other product areas, it was easy to expand the scope of the existing institution to cover medical devices.

Expansion came during the 1930s. W. G. Campbell, the chief of the FDA, and Rexford G. Tugwell, the newly appointed assistant secretary of agriculture, decided to rewrite the legislation in the spring of 1933.[52] A 1933 report by the FDA first raised the problems related to medical devices.

> Mechanical devices, represented as helpful in the cure of disease, may be harmful. Many of them serve a useful and definite purpose. The weak and ailing furnish a fertile field, however, for mechanical devices represented as potent in the treatment of many conditions for which there is no effective mechanical cure. The need for legal control of devices of this type is self-evident. Products and devices intended to effect changes in the physical structure of the body not necessarily associated with disease are extremely prevalent and, in some instances, capable of extreme harm. They are at this time almost wholly beyond the control of any Federal statute. . . . The new statute, if enacted, will bring such products under the jurisdiction of the law.[53]

An interesting evolution in the FDA's orientation from its earlier conception had begun. The FDA moved from the aegis of agriculture, where food was a primary focus, to the Department of Health, Education, and Welfare (HEW), which was concerned with broader issues of health. This shift made device regulation a logical extension of FDA jurisdiction.

Problems of definition arose, however, in the debates over terminology. In early drafts of the 1906 law, drugs were defined more broadly. There was an effort to capture within the regulatory definition both those products used for the diagnosis of disease and products that were clearly fraudulent, such as antifat and reducing potions that did not purport to treat recognized diseases. Some legislators proposed to include therapeutic devices within the definition of drugs. In Senate hearings on the bill, the FDA chief stated that adding medical devices to the

definition of drugs was intended to extend the scope of the law
to include not only products like sutures and surgical dressings
but also "trusses or any other mechanical appliance that might
be employed for the treatment of disease or intended for the
cure or prevention of disease."[54]

The legislative debates on the definition are enlightening, not
for the quality of the debates per se but for their focus. Indeed,
the discussion of the device/drug distinction emerged in a con-
fused context. While Senator Copeland, a major supporter of
the bill, spoke to an amendment of the drug definition to include
drugs used for "diagnosis" of disease as well as for "cure, mitigation, or treatment," his colleague, Senator Clark, objected to the
use of the term *drug* to describe a device. Senator Clark stated
that he did not oppose devices being covered by the law, but to
treat them as drugs "in law and in logic and in lexicography is a
palpable absurdity."[55] Because he was raising an issue not relevant to the amendment under debate, the matter was not resolved at that time. However, Senator Copeland had no fundamental objection to separate definitions, and the later versions
included a separate paragraph defining devices.

Subsequent events made this a very significant distinction
indeed. The first bill was introduced in Congress in 1933 and did
not become law in the subsequent five-year period. The bill
finally got attention following a drug disaster. The Massengill
Company, a drug firm, wanted to sell a liquid form of sulfanilamide, one of the new classes of sulfa drugs on the market
in tablet form. The company dissolved the drug in a chemical
solution and marketed it as Elixir Sulfanilamide in September
1937. The chemical solution, diethylene glycol, was toxic; over
one hundred people died from the elixir. The FDA exercised its
power to seize as much of the preparation as it could find and
managed to retrieve most of it. However, the agency did not
have the power to prosecute Massengill for causing the deaths; it
could only cite them for failing to label the solution properly.
The fine imposed for mislabeling was $26,100.[56]

Public pressure for greater FDA authority arose after this
incident. The pending legislation expanded the FDA's power to
screen all "new drugs" before they could be marketed. This
distinction created a new class of drugs quite separate from

medical devices. The concept of premarket control provided more protection for the consumer than prior labeling and information requirements.

However, this extension of power to regulate "new drugs" had an additional effect on medical devices. They were now included in the final version of the law, but because they were defined separately, the new drug provision did not apply to them. Device producers were subject only to the adulteration and labeling requirements under the law. The emphasis of the lawmakers continued to be on fraudulent devices, not on control of legitimate devices that might have both therapeutic benefit and harmful characteristics.

The FDA's procedural powers over devices were limited to seizure of the misbranded product and prosecution of the producer. It could not initiate regulatory action until a device had entered interstate commerce and then only if it deemed the product improperly labeled ("misbranded") or dangerous ("adulterated").[57] Once the FDA considered a product misbranded or adulterated, it could initiate a seizure action and seek to enjoin the manufacturer from further production of the device.

Seizure was the tactic most frequently employed against device producers in subsequent years. The agency had to file a libel action in a district court, alleging a device to be in violation of the law. The FDA seized the devices before trial. The seizure was upheld only if the FDA could prove its charges at trial. The proceeding affected the specific device seized. Only after the agency succeeded in the initial action could it make multiple seizures or move the court to enjoin further production. Of course, multiple seizures were impractical because it was extremely difficult to trace the ultimate location of the condemned devices and virtually impossible to seize them all. Device manufacturers could evade injunction by making insignificant changes in their products and marketing them as "new devices."[58] The number of trials for fraudulent devices remained small and affected only quack producers at the margins of the industry.

When the federal government addressed problems with medical devices, its powers were limited to procedures which had been inadequate for the regulation of harmful drugs. Despite these problems, however, the 1938 law did set an important precedent. A large, popular federal institution existed to protect the public from harmful products used for health purposes. Devices were generally ignored for nearly forty years, while federal power over the drug marketplace expanded from 1938 to 1962. Not until 1976 did the FDA get jurisdiction to regulate some devices as stringently as new drugs.

Government and Device Distribution

As we have seen, government institutions, primarily the NIH and the FDA, were in place to intervene in the discovery phase of the medical device innovation process. However, the entry of government into the distribution phase lagged behind these developments.

At the beginning of the twentieth century, not much health care was available for the consumer to buy. As we have seen, doctors had a very limited arsenal of treatment options. There were few drugs and fewer medical devices. There was only a primitive understanding of the biological processes of the human body and little that a doctor could do to alleviate illness. Hospitals were used only by the "deserving" poor, who could not be cared for at home but were not candidates for the almshouse. The dismal conditions in hospitals between 1870 and 1920 have been exhaustively documented.[59]

The public sector played only a minor role in support of hospital care. Local governments often supported public hospitals, and some private institutions received local aid. There were no other sources of public funds for hospitals. Although suffering financial woes, a New York City hospital in 1904 would not seek federal support, "No one, in those days, proposed going hat in hand to Albany or Washington."[60]

There were no intermediaries in the costs of sickness for anyone who was not destitute. In the first decades of the twentieth century, Europe began to provide state aid for sickness insurance, but there was no government action to subsidize voluntary expenditures in the United States.[61] There were some progressive reformers that advocated health insurance, both private and public, as early as 1912. However, employers strongly opposed insurance schemes, as did the physicians and labor unions. The medical profession vigorously decried a health insurance referendum in California, alleging that the proposal was linked to sinister forces in Germany.[62]

However, important developments in diagnosis and treatment began to change the attitude of the public toward the desirability of health care. The advent of aseptic surgery and the X-ray machine gave the ill some hope that surgery could cure them. The number of hospitals grew, from 4,000 in 1909 to 7,000 in 1928, and the number of hospital beds expanded from 400,000 to 900,000 as a result. Costs of care began to rise as well. These costs were associated with some new capital equipment, including European innovations for diagnosis and the growth of laboratories.

Unfortunately, the depression in the 1930s meant declines in visits to doctors and hospitals and a consequent drop in the incomes of physicians. Hospitals suffered financially, and at the same time demand increased for free services. Some public welfare payments for medical care were seen as a temporary solution; these continued after the depression.

Important changes were occurring in the market for medical care, but they did not extend to acceptance of federal and state involvement in that market. People had begun to see the value of health care. The middle class no longer was satisfied with attention from the family physician, and the hospital offered important services not available at home. At the same time medical science held out hope, however, the depression made health care inaccessible to large numbers of Americans. There was a perceived need for more health care, but few resources were available to pay for it. Pressure for greater access, particularly by the middle class, would ultimately bring the government into the marketplace. However, the idea of government subsidies met with considerable resistance, and health care took a back seat to other pressing social needs, such as public assistance and welfare.

As America emerged from the Great Depression and approached World War II, significant changes had occurred in the relationship between government and innovation. The NIH was established to promote basic medical science research, which indirectly affected the medical device industry. The federal government also had made significant steps toward direct regulation of product producers in the 1938 Food, Drug, and Cosmetic Act. The government had not, as yet, committed itself to payment for health care. This development lay ahead.

WORLD WAR II ACCELERATES INTERACTION

As the nation mobilized for war in the 1940s, the federal government became involved in many activities previously left to the private sector. Government leadership in the war effort changed the public perception about its basic role in science and medicine.

Wartime Innovation

The federal government had an effect on all stages of the innovation process in medical devices during the war. Government spending promoted basic science as well as technological invention and development. Government also became a major consumer of both medical technology and military technology, greatly expanding the market for products produced by firms with medical technology expertise.

President Roosevelt established the Office of Scientific Research and Development (OSRD) in 1941, and it had two parallel committees on national defense and medical research. The Committee on Medical Research (CMR) mounted a comprehensive program to address medical problems associated with the war. The government gave 450 contracts to universities and 150 more to research institutes, hospitals, and other organizations. In total, the office spent $15 million and involved some 5,500 scientists and technicians. Government supported achievements included a synthetic atabrine for malaria treatment (which replaced the quinine seized by Japan), therapeutically useful derivatives of blood, and the development of penicillin.[63]

The OSRD was unique because it was organized as an independent civilian enterprise and managed by academic and industrial scientists in equal partnership with the military. In contrast with World War I, where scientists served as military officers under military commanders, the work of OSRD was fully funded by the government, but scientists worked in their own institutional settings. The research contract model proved to be a flexible instrument in the subsequent partnership between government and private institutions during the postwar period.[64]

Government also let contracts for development of wartime technologies. Some of these efforts benefited device companies directly because they had technologies that could be channeled for military use. Other government efforts promoted technologies that would later prove useful in medical device technology. In addition, the government was a ready market for military and medical supplies. Government purchasing enriched many companies in the instrument business, such as Beckman and GE. Government policy helped to establish a technology base for postwar development and allowed firms to take advantage of the postwar boom.

In addition, federal government spending and greater need for health care for service personnel injured in combat stimulated the medical technology market. The federal government provided medical services for all military personnel—60 percent of all hospital beds were used by the military. Thus government also became a large consumer of medical supplies and equipment.

Medical Device Successes in Wartime

The war provided an impetus to innovation in medical device technology. Three profiles of successful firms—Beckman Instruments, Baxter Travenol, and General Electric—illustrate the effect of government on innovation.

Beckman

Beckman Instruments provides an excellent example of the impact of the war on medical device technology. The National Technical Laboratories, as the firm was called at the time, did not make weapons but did make important military products. Its contribution to the war effort is reflected in sales data: gross sales were thirty-four times larger in 1950 than in 1940.

One key product was Beckman's "Helipot," a unique instrument for use in radar systems. The U.S. military requested meters built to military specifications for the radar program and able to withstand strong mechanical shocks. Beckman recalled, "I began to get calls from lieutenants and captains and finally from generals and admirals. There were ships that couldn't sail because they didn't have Helipots for their radars."[65] Beckman himself redesigned the instrument. In the first year of production, the new model accounted for 40 percent of the firm's total profits.

Because wartime disrupted supplies of essential products, new markets opened and creativity was welcomed and rewarded. Beckman's spectrophotometer, which used a quartz prism and a newly developed light source and phototube, is a good example. This model, introduced in 1941, could accurately measure the vitamin content of a substance. The war had cut off the supply of cod liver oil, which was a rich source of vitamins A and D, from Scandinavia. Before the Beckman instrument, there was no way to efficiently measure the vitamin content of other foods to plan healthy diets. The Beckman spectrophotometer determined vitamin content precisely in one or two minutes.

Rubber supplies had been cut off by the bombing of Pearl Harbor, and the nation desperately needed a substitute. Supported by the federal Office of Rubber Reserve, Beckman developed infrared spectrophotometers that could detect butadiene, a major ingredient in synthetic rubber. Later on, Beckman was also involved in a government project with the Massachusetts Institute of Technology, working under the Atomic Energy Commission, to develop a recording instrument to monitor radioactivity levels in atomic energy plants.

These new technologies frequently proved to have medical applications. With friends from the California Institute of Technology, Beckman produced oxygen meters for the navy. An anesthesiologist heard about the meter in its development stage and was interested in its use to measure oxygen in infant incubators. If oxygen supplies to a baby are too low, the infant will not thrive; if oxygen levels are too high, it can become blind. This doctor treated his own grandchild with a Beckman meter, feeding oxygen from a tank into a cardboard box and thereby saving the baby's life. However, during the war, hospitals could not afford oxygen meters. It was twelve years later that hospitals began to purchase them in large numbers.

Baxter Travenol

Baxter Travenol provides another wartime success story. Although the medical theory underlying intravenous (IV) therapy was clearly understood at the outset of the twentieth century, only large research and teaching hospitals could prepare solutions and equipment properly. Even carefully prepared solutions caused adverse reactions, such as severe chills and fevers, because pyrogens produced by bacteria remained in the solutions after sterilization.

In 1931, Idaho surgeon Ralph Falk, his brother, and Dr. Donald Baxter believed they could eliminate the pyrogen problem through controlled production in evacuated containers. When reactions continued to occur in patients, the doctors discovered that pyrogens were present in the rubber infusion equipment used by hospitals. They used disposable plastic tubing to eliminate this source of bacteria and worked with a glass manufacturer to produce a coating that resisted the contamination caused by the deterioration of the bottles that held the solutions.

In 1939 the fledgling company pioneered another medical breakthrough—a container for blood collection and storage. It was the first sterile, pyrogen-free, vacuum-type blood unit for indirect transfusion. It allowed storage of blood products for up to twenty-one days, making blood banking practical for the first time. The enormous demand for IV equipment and blood transfusions during World War II was a boon for Baxter. Its solutions were the only ones approved for wartime use by the U.S. military. Sales dropped dramatically after the war and rose again several years later during the Korean War. These fluctuating fortunes stabilized, and twenty-five years of uninterrupted company growth occurred after 1955 onward.[66]

General Electric

General Electric was involved in every facet of the war, including building engines for planes, tanks, ships, and submarines. It provided electrical capacity for large-scale manufacturing and also built power plants, testing equipment, and radio equipment.[67] GE's activities extended to medical care for combat forces. Innovation was integral to that effort, as well as to the engines of war. "All along the story was the same. The war production job was one of prodigious quantities of all kinds of equipment. But it was also a job of constantly seeking ways to improve that equipment. Only the best was good enough, and the best today might be second best next week."[68]

General Electric's war-inspired medical equipment innovations included portable X-ray machines for use on ships and relatively inaccessible stations such as Pacific island hospitals. X-ray machines were also used to screen inductees for tuberculosis, and GE created cost-saving features, including machines that used smaller films. In addition, it built refrigeration and air-conditioning systems for blood and penicillin storage. Government purchasing expanded market size. The army bought hundreds of electrocardiograph machines, ultraviolet lamps, and devices for diagnosis and therapy treatments.[69]

The war affected innovation in dramatic ways. At the discovery stage, medical device innovation was stimulated and encouraged. Many technological innovations in materials science, radar, ultrasound, and other advancements had significant medical implications in the postwar period. Government purchasing stimulated the distribution of devices as well. The number of device producers and the value of their shipments grew in every SIC code.

Just as important, but less visible, were the institutional changes that occurred. Before the war, major public institutions had been formed that presaged government intervention in the discovery phase, most notably the NIH and the FDA. Wartime demands also accelerated the general public's acceptance of government involvement in scientific research and new technology. All these forces led to significant government activity in all phases of medical device innovation. The patient soon received extensive treatment.

PART TWO
THE TREATMENT

GLENDOWER: I can call spirits from the vasty
                        deep.
HOTSPUR: Why, so can I, or so can any man,
                        But will they come when you do
                        call for them?

I Henry IV III.i. 51–53

3

GOVERNMENT PROMOTES MEDICAL
DEVICE DISCOVERY

	Discovery	Distribution
Promote	1. National Institutes of Health (NIH) Space & Defense Spinoffs	2. Hill-Burton Hospital Construction Funds Medicare/Medicaid
Inhibit	3. Regulation (FDA) Product Liability	4. Certificate of Need Cost-Containment Technology Assessment

Figure 6. The policy matrix.

After World War II, the federal government was firmly committed to supporting for basic scientific research. Indeed, government came to be seen as a legitimate vehicle for the promotion of innovation. The issue was no longer whether government should provide research and development (R&D) support, but to whom, how much, and in what form. Three primary areas of federal research emerged—defense, space, and civilian, the last dominated by biomedical science. (See figure 6.) There is constant political debate about the overall size of the federal R&D pie and the allocation of funds among these various programs.[1]

Research and development support can take several forms— federal money for basic science research, federal funds directed or targeted toward specific technologies or products, and federal incentives for institutional transfer of technology from basic science to commercialization. The federal government has provided all three forms to biomedical research, each with the potential to affect the medical device industry. Figure 7 illustrates how the forms of funding related to the innovation continuum.

Federal R&D dollars have affected medical device innovation at various points on the innovation continuum. This chapter discusses the evolution of various policies to support medical device discovery. The first, and most significant, policy involves grants for basic science research through the National Institutes of Health. The second, introduced in the 1960s, targets specific technologies at the point of invention and development. The Artificial Heart Program (AHP) at the NIH illustrates this form of support. Medical device discovery has benefited from spinoffs of targeted programs for space and defense purposes, and these programs are discussed as well. Finally, this chapter describes congressional policies to facilitate technology transfer—from universities, government laboratories, and private firms. The goal of these policies is to rectify perceived institutional barriers to progress along the innovation continuum.

GOVERNMENT SUPPORT FOR BASIC SCIENCE

When Congress promoted health research after the war, the NIH was the logical federal institution to administer it. Congress both enlarged the authority of the NIH and provided increasingly generous funding for it. The Public Health Service Act of 1944 extended NIH research authority from cancer to health and disease generally.[2] In 1948, the National Heart Institute and the National Dental Institute were established, and the name of the agency officially changed to the National Institutes of Health to reflect the categorical or disease oriented approach of the multi-institute structure. The total congressional appropriation rose from $7 million in 1947 to $70 million by 1952.[3] By 1955, the NIH awarded 3,300 research grants and 1,900 training grants, accounting for over 70 percent of the NIH budget.[4] President Kennedy, a strong supporter of the NIH, included in his first budget an increase of $40 million, the largest increase ever for medical research and the largest percentage raise since 1955. The rationale for this rapid expansion was "an expanding economy, a favorable political ambience, a consensus stemming

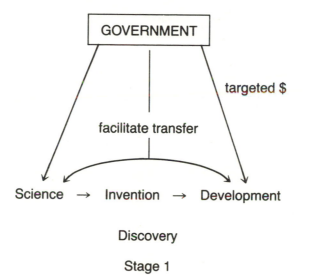

Figure 7. Forms of government support for biomedical R&D.

largely from World War II technological success that scientific research can pay off big, and a set of remarkably effective health leaders in both public and private sectors."[5]

The primary form or strategy of support has been called the "boiling soup" concept. The investigator-initiated grant process allowed scientists to work on many projects. Essentially undirected, individual investigators each followed his or her own path of discovery. This philosophy was well articulated in the Senate Appropriations Committee Report on the Labor-HEW Appropriation Bill for 1967.

> The committee continues to be convinced that progress of medical knowledge is basically dependent upon full support of undirected basic and applied research effort of scientists working individually or in groups on the ideas, problems, and purposes of their selection and judged by their scientific peers to be scientifically meaningful, excellent, and relevant to extending knowledge of human health and disease.[6]

Congress maintained a hands-off approach and "tiptoed lightly so as not to disturb genius at work."[7]

Certain institutional patterns emerged as a result. Support flowed from the NIH to researchers engaged in basic science at universities and medical schools. The NIH had an enormous influence on the research environment. Research became the major, if not the dominant, feature in academic medicine, and a partnership between universities and government scientists developed. As government came to provide virtually all of the resources for academic research, these institutions thrived on the largesse.[8] By 1979, the NIH provided over 40 percent of all health R&D funds (see figure 8). This strategy forged a very strong philosophical and institutional link between the NIH and academic medicine.

While basic science in the academic research community received the bulk of NIH funds, Congress increased the role of small business in federally sponsored research through the Small Business Innovation Development Act of 1982. The act created the Small Business Innovation and Research Program (SBIR), the goal of which is to support small firms in early stages of research with the expectation that they will ultimately attract private capital and commercialize their results. A small, fixed percentage of all research funds must be directed toward small businesses under the law, and eleven federal agencies are required to participate. The NIH accounts for 92 percent of the SBIR projects within the Department of Health and Human Services and devoted $61.6 million to the program in fiscal year 1987.[9]

SBIR proposals are investigator initiated and reviewed through traditional NIH mechanisms. Some successes have emerged from the program. For example, two current commercial devices resulted from SBIR funding—a laser that removes certain birthmarks known as port-wine stains and an electrode that can be swallowed to use in emergency cardiac pacing.[10]

That support for basic scientific research leads to advances in medicine is not in question. In a well-known study, Comroe and Dripps found that basic research provided a critical influence in the long road leading to clinical applications and technology useful in patient care.[11] While direct links are often difficult to demonstrate, the general consensus can be summed up in the following manner.

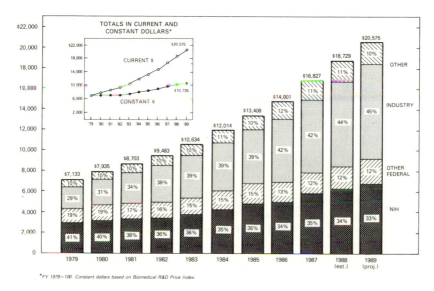

Figure 8. National support for health R&D by source, 1979–1989 (in millions of dollars).
Source: NIH Data Book, no. 90–1261 (December 1989).

Although innovation in pharmaceuticals and medical devices has been largely generated in the private sector by private research and investment, it is doubtful whether much of this would have taken place without the base of knowledge resulting from government-sponsored programs. Much modern medical instrumentation and diagnostics derive from basic advances in the physical sciences, including laboratory instrumentation, which occurred as a result of broad-based government sponsorship of fundamental physics, chemistry, and biology.[12]

How is the information developed in these laboratories transferred to industry? Academic journals are the traditional outlet for scientific findings. Academic researchers are rewarded for publishing the results of their scientific work. This information is in the public domain, and scientists, engineers, and entrepreneurs interested in product development acquire this information and apply it to their own projects. Thus, federal funds only indirectly support product development, depending on the initiative of private firms.

Scientific journals can be an inefficient means of transferring technology. Delays in publication and the multiplicity of articles affect the speed and completeness of information acquisition. Efficiency of transfer can be complicated for medical devices, the development of which may depend on information from many disciplines with data contained in a wide variety of journals and specialties.

The focus of NIH support on basic science created institutional limitations for medical device development. First, there tends to be an anti-engineering bias at the NIH. Unlike biochemical research, such as studies of organ function or disease processes, medical device innovation is multidisciplinary and may require a confluence of engineering disciplines and materials sciences as well as biochemistry, medicine, and biology. Indeed, as recently as 1987, a committee of the National Research Council concluded that bioengineering studies accounted for only about 3 percent of the NIH extramural research budget. This low figure may reflect either a lack of applicant interest or, more likely, a lack of receptivity by NIH committees, given that few engineers participate in ranking and funding decisions.[13]

Thus, although it may be difficult to pinpoint direct cause and effect, medical device innovation was probably assisted in general by the growing expertise in fundamental scientific understanding of the human body and disease processes that the NIH policies encouraged. However, a government policy biased toward biochemistry may have disadvantaged the engineering based medical device industry, at least relative to other forms of biomedical research.

DIRECT TARGETING OF MEDICAL DEVICE TECHNOLOGIES

Several events occurred in the 1960s that fostered changes in the NIH research focus. Increased scientific understanding of disease led to more and better options for medical care. That created public clamor for greater access to these new treatments. In 1966, Congress enacted the Medicare and Medicaid programs for the elderly, disabled, and indigent, which are discussed at greater length in chapter 4. Members of Congress could then point to support for medical services as evidence of their concern for the public's health. Spending for services became more popular than basic science research, the results of which are long-term and difficult to document.

To the extent that Congress supported R&D, the pressure was for "results not research," as President Johnson so aptly put it.[14] There was growing public concern in the mid-sixties for the NIH to justify its size and its mission. Congress saw the success of the space program, with its targeted and focused goals, as a model for solving technological challenges in health research. The result was increased political pressure for more federal control of research through targeted programs with specific goals.

In the next few years, Congress established NIH programs modeled upon a systems approach to innovation. The Artificial Heart Program (AHP) in the National Heart Institute (NHI), the Artificial Kidney (AK-CU) Program in the National Institute of Arthritis and Metabolic Diseases, and aspects of Nixon's War on Cancer are three of the better-known targeted projects.[15] Mission oriented research also included the creation of large centers with groups of investigators performing government designed research and clinical trials. By the 1970s, mission oriented research comprised almost 40 percent of the NHI's budget, although other institutes retained a stronger commitment to the traditional model of investigator-initiated grants.

The Artificial Heart Program illustrates the institutional adjustments required for the NIH to manage technology development in a targeted program. It also highlights the politics of federal R&D as Congress tangled with scientists over the creation and continuation of the program.

The Artificial Heart Program

In order to understand the political appeal of developing an artificial heart, one must know something about cardiology. Heart failure is the most common disorder leading to loss of health or life. In theory, an artificial replacement heart can prevent the threat of imminent death from end-stage heart disease. Early estimates of the number of patients who might benefit from an artificial heart were as high as 130,000 per year.[16]

The heart functions mechanically, rather than through a primarily chemical or electrochemical process as the kidney and liver do. Far more than other vital organs, the heart is inherently suitable for replacement by a mechanical device. Scientific work on the concept had been underway in several laboratories in the 1950s. Researchers knew that they had to design a pump, an engine to drive it, and a power source. The challenge was to find materials to line the pump that would not injure the blood and a substance for the heart itself that was flexible and durable enough to withstand the constant squeezing and relaxing motions. All the parts needed to be synchronized to sustain life.[17] (See figure 9.)

Scientists were divided on the feasibility or desirability of artificial hearts; the NIH was unlikely to have funded proposals to work on the technology. The most enthusiastic supporters were some heart surgeons, notably Dr. Michael DeBakey. Congress, unlike the NIH scientists, was receptive because of the political salience of the project. As noted above, many Americans feared death from heart disease, and efforts to eliminate the disease were popular. The idea captured the imagination of Congress and fit the new notion of results oriented research. The successes of the space program were an added impetus. Recently, Dr. DeBakey pointedly recalled the political situation. "Jim Shannon [the NIH director] was opposed to the concept and NIH's involvement in it because he thought there was not enough basic knowledge and that it was not scientifically sound. I went over his head, to Congress."[18]

As a result, Congress studied the feasibility of the project. It established the Artificial Heart Program in July 1964 with an initial appropriation of $581,000. The program was housed in the National Heart, Lung, and Blood Institute (NHLBI), the successor to the old NHI.

Targeted programs like the AHP challenged the relationship between academic medicine and the NIH. The program, freed from the traditional concepts of NIH basic research, was much more open to engineering and to industry. Development of the artificial heart required technological expertise not found in medical schools or university science departments; engineers and private firms had to be included.[19]

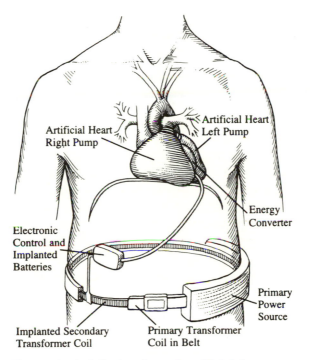

Figure 9. A fully implanted artificial heart system.

Source: Artificial Heart and Assist Devices: Directions, Needs, Costs, Societal and Ethical Issues, NIH publication no. 85–2723 (May 1985), 11.

The NIH needed new tools and procedures to implement targeted programs. The National Cancer Institute (NCI), under Dr. Kenneth Endicott, had pioneered the use of the contract, despite considerable objections from more traditional scientists. The contract form allowed the professional staff at the NCI to specify what research it desired, to solicit proposals from interested researchers in business and academics, and to choose who would undertake the proposed project.

The use of the contract also appeared in the early days of the AHP. Dr. John R. Beem, director of the AHP, came from industry. He assembled a small staff familiar with systems approaches, including experts associated with NASA and the air force. Because of the technological requirements, the NIH sought special permission to consider contracts rather than grants and, in 1964, let nine contracts which were among their first nondrug contracts. They covered such goals as the development of pumps, drive units, mock circulating systems, and blood-compatible materials. The early contracts were with medical engineering teams at various large industrial firms, such as Westinghouse and SRI, none of which were traditional NIH partners. Contracts with small innovators later became the norm.[20]

These contracts with industry were controversial within the NIH, primarily because they threatened the traditional partnership with universities. Some NIH leaders did not enthusiastically support contracts. They "did not take kindly . . . to the idea of taking large amounts of research money and funneling them to profit-making industrial firms through the targeted contract mechanism."[21] Conflicts between engineers and medical scientists arose. One chronicler of the program wrote:

> The two disciplines, medicine and the scientific art, and engineering with its underpinnings in the physical sciences, could not always fulfill each other's expectations. The NHI emphasis was naturally on the medical researcher and the clinical investigator and their needs; the engineers were often treated as "hardware kids" and many marriages between teams at hospital centers and industrial laboratories ended in divorce.[22]

The program has been steeped in politics throughout its twenty-five years. Congressional enthusiasm began to wane in the late 1960s when results were not immediately forthcoming, but support has persisted, albeit at modest levels. Within a few years of its inception, the program expenditures had increased to approximately $10 million. Since 1975, expenditures have stabilized in the range of $10 to $12 million annually. This amount represents only about 1 percent of the NHLBI budget. The total expenditures to 1988 have been about $240 million.

The most recent political conflict over the program occurred in 1988, when a small group of senators forced Dr. Claude Lenfant, director of the NHLBI, to reconsider a proposal to restructure the Artificial Heart Program. Lenfant had suspended financing for research on totally implantable hearts, choosing to focus instead on development of LVADs, or left ventricle assist devices, which help but do not replace the diseased heart. The NIH capitulated; the *New York Times* reported that Lenfant's superiors, "fearing that all of their future programs would be in jeopardy, forced him to 'eat a little crow.'"[23]

There is a contentious debate about the wisdom of the AHP, with critics questioning both the costs of the technology and the ethics of the research. Twenty-five years after the program began, a viable artificial organ has not yet been produced. Some of the ethical and social issues raised by this program, and its relationship with other sources of public policy, are discussed in chapters 9 and 10. Without engaging in the debate at this point, we can reflect on the benefits of this and other similar programs for medical device innovation.

For companies in the industry, the benefits of targeted device development are clear. The AHP broke down some of the traditional barriers to bioengineering that had developed within the NIH. The agency began to interact with firms as well as university scientists, reducing institutional and disciplinary barriers for applied bioengineering projects. Thus, medical device innovators have been included in, but are clearly only a small part of, the mission of the NIH.

MEDICAL DEVICE SPINOFFS FROM SPACE AND DEFENSE RESEARCH

Anyone who has spent time in a hospital is aware of the array of equipment used to monitor a patient's condition. Many patients may not know that the needs of astronauts contributed to this technology. Patients undergoing a noninvasive ultrasound diagnosis are probably unaware that it was the navy's search for tools to detect enemy submarines that generated understanding of this technology. Similarly, the intensive search for military uses for lasers has brought us promising treatments for cataracts and cancerous tumors.

How did these space and defense technologies arrive in our health care system? Obviously, the space and defense programs do not focus on medicine; they have other specific missions to accomplish. Through a variety of ways, however, medical technologies have developed from research in these nonmedical, government sponsored programs.

Medical Applications of Space Technologies

Sputnik, the USSR's successful satellite launched in late 1957, alarmed Americans who assumed that the United States was losing technological competitiveness to the Soviets. The U.S. space program was a direct response. By early 1958, Congress had introduced numerous bills; President Eisenhower signed the National Aeronautics and Space Act in July 1958.[24]

The National Aeronautics and Space Administration (NASA) had to consolidate a number of projects and personnel from government and recast the former National Advisory Committee on Aeronautics (NACA). NACA had engaged in in-house research entirely and had little experience in developing and implementing large-scale projects.[25] NASA became a contracting agency; 90 percent of its annual expenditures by 1962 went for goods and services procured by outside contractors.

From the beginning, NASA was a public relations tool for the United States. Not only was it designed to win the space race, but also it let everyone know that the U.S. had restaked its claim to be the world leader in technology. To this end, NASA was to "provide the widest practicable and appropriate dissemination of information concerning its activities and the results thereof."[26] NASA's survival depended on success in its mission and public perception that the program was worthwhile. Thus NASA had to fight to establish and maintain its legitimacy.

NASA's first decade was successful in terms of government and popular support. Following the launch of the *Apollo* and the moon landing in 1969, however, enthusiasm for the program waned. During NASA's second decade, its total budget fell. President Nixon urged NASA to turn its attention to solving practical problems on earth, and funding dedicated to promoting civilian applications of NASA supported technology rose.[27] Toward the end of the 1970s, Congress created NASA's Technology Utilization Program, which included regional technology transfer experts. Their job was to monitor R&D contracts to ensure that new technology, whether developed in-house or by contractors, would be available for secondary use. In addition, NASA opened a number of user-assistance centers to provide information retrieval services and technical help to industrial and government entities. NASA characterizes itself as a national resource providing "a bank of technical knowledge available for reuse."[28] By 1985, NASA claimed an estimated 30,000 secondary applications of aerospace technology.

Many of the systems developed for the space program have medical applications. The technology tends to derive from NASA's needs for super-efficient, yet small and light, technologies and its need to monitor the vital signs and overall health of astronauts in space. Technology transfer to medicine has occurred in several ways. NASA contractors form new companies to market products that are based on technology developed for NASA. Sometimes large firms form medically related subsidiaries subsequent to completion of a NASA contract. On occasion, companies with no prior relationship with the agency approach NASA to acquire the technology necessary for the development of a medical product. In all cases, NASA encourages the transfer of technology to civilian uses.

For example, NASA needed new technology to meet the challenges of monitoring the astronauts' vital signs. The commonly used conducting electrode was attached to the body through a paste electrolyte. This method could not be used for long-term monitoring because the paste dries and causes distortions of the data. Other electrodes that made direct contact without use of paste electrolyte failed because body movements caused signal-distorting noise as well. NASA contracted with Texas Technical University scientists who developed an advanced electrocardiographic electrode. It was constructed of a thin dielectric (non-conducting) film applied to a stainless steel surface. It functioned immediately on contact with the skin and was not affected by ambient conditions of temperature, light, or moisture. NASA was assigned the patent and subsequently awarded a license for its use to a California entrepreneur who founded Heart Rate, Inc. The small firm has continued to develop and produce heart rate monitors for medical markets.[29]

The Q-Med firm produced another monitoring product from

electrode technology developed at NASA's Johnson Space Center. Q-Med received an exclusive license from NASA to manufacture and market electrodes in 1984. The firm's monitor assists ambulatory patients who have coronary artery disease and can be worn for days, months, or years to evaluate every heartbeat. It stores information for later review by a physician, who can program it for specific cardiac conditions. The monitor can summon immediate aid if the wearer experiences abnormal heartbeats.[30]

NASA also needed information about spacecraft conditions. For example, McDonnell Douglas Corporation, a firm with many NASA contracts, developed a device to detect bacterial contamination in a space vehicle. In another contract, it developed additional capabilities to detect and identify bacterial infections among the crew of a manned mission to Mars. McDonnell Douglas formed the Vitek subsidiary to manufacture and market a system known as the AutoMicrobic System (AMS). The system, introduced in 1979, offered rapid identification and early treatment of infection. AMS provides results in four to thirteen hours; conventional culture preparations take from two to four days.[31]

The confinements of the small spacecraft created a need for miniaturized products. NASA developed a portable X-ray instrument that is now produced as a medical system. The lixiscope, or *low intensity* X-ray *imaging* scope, is a self-contained, battery-powered fluoroscope that produces an instant image through use of a small amount of radioactive isotope. It uses less than 1 percent of the radiation required by conventional X-ray devices and can be used in emergency field situations and in dental and orthopedic surgery.[32] Lixi acquired an exclusive NASA license to produce one version of the device.

NASA awarded a contract to Parker Hannifin Corporation, one of the world's primary suppliers of fluid system components, to develop and produce equipment for controlling the flow of propellants into the engines of the *Saturn* moonbooster. It subsequently has worked on many other space projects, including miniaturized systems. In 1977, Parker's aerospace group formed a biomedical products division to apply aerospace technology, particularly miniaturized fluid control technology, to medical devices. Products include a continuous, computer directed system to deliver medication. Parker's key contributions were a tiny pump capable of metering medication to target organs in precise doses, an external programmable medication device for external use, and a plasma filtration system that removes from the blood certain substances believed to contribute to the progression of diseases such as rheumatoid arthritis and lupus.[33]

Another application has been an implantable, programmable medication system that meters the flow of drugs. The electronic system delivers programmed medication by wireless telemetry— a space technology—in which command signals are sent to the implanted device by means of a transmitting antenna. Precise monitoring of drugs can be a godsend to a patient. Such a system allows for constant levels of medication, avoiding the highs and lows caused by administering injections at set intervals. Targeting drugs to specific organs makes dosages more accurate and avoids exposing the whole body to toxic therapeutic agents. Some of this research involves cooperative efforts by NASA, universities, and private firms. The Applied Physics Lab at Johns Hopkins University and the Goddard Space Flight Center offer program management and technical expertise. Medical equipment companies, including Pacesetter, provide part of the funding and produce these systems for the commercial market.[34]

The NASA experience offers some important lessons. NASA has demonstrated that there is no inherent conflict in government, universities, and industries working together to create useful medical products. It has also shown, on a limited scale and within its particular mission, that government supported R&D can be effectively transferred to the private sector. The benefits to the medical device industry have been important, albeit small relative to NASA's overall expenditures.

Medical Applications of Defense Technologies

Spending on military R&D has been a high priority and accounts for nearly half of all federal R&D. Important medical technologies have emerged from defense research, and the stories of ultrasound and lasers illustrate the potential, as well as the limitations, of medical spinoffs from defense related R&D.

Ultrasound

Ultrasound is a mechanical vibration at high frequencies above the range of human hearing. In 1880, Pierre and Jacques Curie discovered what is known as the *piezoelectric effect*, in which an electric charge is produced in response to pressure on such materials as quartz. Conversely, mechanical deformation results from an applied voltage. The impact of sound waves producing this mechanical deformation can be transformed into electrical energy and recorded. Devices to generate and to detect ultrasonic energy are derived from this discovery.[35]

World War I led to the first efforts to develop large-scale practical applications of this physical concept. The French government commissioned a physicist to use high-frequency ultrasound to detect submarines underwater. These efforts, conducted in cooperation with Britain and the United States, continued throughout the war. No practical results were achieved at the time, but work continued between the wars. The Naval Research Laboratory refined the basic technology using new electronic techniques and studied the qualities of underwater sound. Scientists also studied industrial applications, including the ability to detect otherwise hidden flaws in industrial materials. There were some medical applications, but these were virtually therapeutic rather than diagnostic, based on the controversial concept of irradiating the body to cure diseases.

World War II accelerated research; military sonar (sound navigation and ranging) and radar techniques were based on the echo principle of ultrasound. Virtually all of the later diagnostic applications of ultrasound involved direct contact and/or collaboration with military and industrial personnel and equipment. The war was crucial to the development of the technology.

Industrial and medical applications began to develop in many nations after the war. Dr. George Ludwig was an early American leader who had spent the years from 1947 to 1949 at the Naval Medical Research Institute. He and his collaborators conducted experiments for the navy on the diagnostic capacities of ultra-sound, concentrating on the detection of gallstones. Ludwig acknowledged military research as well as industrial applications as the sources for his investigations.

Dr. John J. Wild, an Englishman familiar with ultrasonic ranging from his wartime experiences, was another early researcher. He came to the United States after World War II. In conjunction with the Wold Chamberlain Naval Air Station, he began experiments to measure tissue thickness. In collaboration with navy engineers, Wild discovered that echoes from tumor-invaded tissue were distinguishable from those produced by normal tissue, establishing the potential for diagnostic applications. Wild later set up research facilities at the University of Minnesota.

Another early pioneer was William J. Fry, a physicist who worked on the design of piezoelectric transducers at the Naval Research Laboratory Underwater Sound Division during the war. He left in 1946, taking his expertise to the University of Illinois where he founded the Bioacoustics Laboratory. In the 1950s, he recognized that high-intensity ultrasound could eventually provide unique advantages to investigating brain mechanisms. In pursuit of these goals, the Office of Naval Research granted him a contract to develop equipment that would pinpoint lesions within the central nervous system of animals.

By the end of the 1950s, ultrasound diagnosis had been introduced into many medical specialties, including neurology, cardiology, gynecology, and ophthalmology. Engineers and physicists, in private industry and in universities, provided the technical design skills to the medical practitioners who understood clinical needs and had access to patients. This fruitful symbiotic relationship continued through the decades as the benefits of ultrasound became more widely recognized. The NIH supported many of the academic research programs from which commercial instruments emerged.[36]

The value of the medical technology was quickly recognized. The procedure was significantly safer than X-rays and could detect certain problems more effectively. The first commercial sales occurred in 1963, and sales held steady at about $1 million a year until the late sixties. They skyrocketed in the 1970s, rising from $10 million in 1973, to $77 million in 1980, to $145 million in 1987.[37]

Lasers

The medical applications for lasers have had a much more complicated development than ultrasound. Laser is an acronym for *l*ight *a*mplification by *s*timulated *e*mission of *r*adiation. The theoretical knowledge to create a laser has been available since the 1920s, but the technical ingredients were not assembled until the 1950s. Pioneers in laser technology include Professors Gordon Gould and Charles Townes, and Arthur Schawlow from Bell Labs. Laser research quickly became the focus of physics, engineering, and optical sciences. Development followed no simple linear sequence. The scientific inquiry, device development, commercialization, and application of system components were parallel occurrences and influenced each other. Lasers represent a family of devices that have each developed and matured at different rates for a wide variety of applications.[38]

A laser requires a lasing medium, or the substance to which energy is applied to create laser light. It must also have an excitation source, or a source of energy, and an optical resonator, which is the chamber where light is held, amplified, and released in a controlled manner. There are a number of types of laser light—it can be continuous or pulsed and have several visible colors or only ultraviolet—and a range of power levels. Types of lasers are named for the lasing medium. For example, there are chemical lasers, lasers with a fiber-optic light source, gas dynamic lasers, such as helium-neon with low-energy beams or carbon dioxide with low- to high-energy beams, and excimer lasers, which produce a high-energy ultraviolet output of gases combined under pressure.

In 1960, between twenty-five and fifty organizations worldwide worked on lasers. Within three years, the number increased to more than five hundred. There were anticipated industrial, military, and medical uses for the technology, and the military provided the most lucrative funds for R&D. In 1963, military funding was $15 million while industry invested only $5 to $10 million, and laser sales at that time were a mere $1 million. Clearly the private market could not sustain the costs of research. Many of the early researchers formed small companies and gravitated to the military. Herbert Dwight, an engineer and founder of Spectra-Physics, commented that "it was relatively easy on an unsolicited proposal to go out and get a relatively nominal contract with somebody like the Naval Research Laboratory . . . a well-known researcher with a good idea could sit down with a top representative of the NRL and pretty much on a word of mouth commitment get money to do work in promising areas."[39]

The Department of Defense, while quite enthusiastic about the potential of lasers, was unsophisticated in early contracts and got very little for its money in some instances. One company, TRG, received about $2 million of federal money and produced comparatively few discoveries. In 1965, a Battelle Memorial Institute report stated that "[the] very high [Department of Defense] budget for [research and development, testing, and evaluation] funds . . . encouraged many small companies to be forced to serve extremely specialized defense markets."[40]

Military funding diverted research from the civilian markets. Consumer oriented firms did not have the resources to invest in long-term R&D. Laser applications in civilian areas stagnated as the Department of Defense directed R&D money to strategic and battlefield weapons, especially during the height of the Vietnam War. The military liked lasers because of their performance superiority over microwave systems. Military R&D focused on very high-powered lasers in the search for "death ray" weapons. Nonmilitary applications required low-powered beams that would not harm human tissue. It can be argued that industrial and medical applications were seriously disadvantaged by the diversion of laser research to military applications.

Thus, many civilian oriented firms floundered. As late as 1987, U.S. manufacturers, as well as European and Japanese firms, struggled to show a profit. These problems are not caused solely by a skewed focus on military applications. The technology has many variations and has advanced rapidly, leaving some companies with outdated systems. There are a wide variety of laser uses, and for any given type there are only a limited number of units produced, so manufacturing costs remain high.[41]

The maturity of the clinical applications varies across medical fields (see figure 10).

However, the civilian laser market, despite its rocky start, still looks promising for medicine in the long term. The most advanced, or mature, area of clinical application is ophthalmic surgery, and many other medical specialties are beginning to use lasers as well. There are promising new applications in cardiovascular surgery, in which research sponsored by the military has played a role. Excimer lasers, developed for the Defense Department at the Jet Propulsion Laboratory,[42] generate short pulses of ultraviolet light that break down the molecules in plaque. Doctors can thread a tiny optical fiber through the artery. The laser probe vaporizes the fatty deposits without damaging surrounding tissue. Before this development, the laser beam sometimes burned a hole in the artery wall or made an opening through the blockage that allowed a clot to form or fatty deposits to rebuild. In early 1987, the FDA approved a laser probe developed by Trimadyne Company.

It has been argued that while defense related R&D has created important spillovers to civilian uses, these occur only in the early stages of development, when "technologies appear to display greater commonality between military and civilian design and performance characteristics. Over time, military and civilian requirements typically diverge, resulting in declining commercial payoffs from military R&D."[43] Indeed, some have suggested that defense R&D may actually interfere with the competitive abilities of firms, citing among other reasons the erosion of some firms' cost discipline as a result of operating in the more insulated competitive environment of military procurement.[44]

In laser research, there have clearly been benefits from military research to the civilian producers. However, the evidence supports the analysis that industrial and medical uses were delayed or disrupted because of diversion of research to military purposes.

Both the space and the defense R&D programs have had spin-off effects for medical devices. However, these benefits have been modest, particularly in relation to the expenditures of the space program, and, in the case of defense research, unpredictable. Without devaluing the benefits, medical science

Embryonic	Growth	Maturity	Decline

SPECIALTY

Estimated Penetration Rates

Ophthalmology	65%
ENT	30%
Gastroenterology	25%
Gynecology	20%
Dermatology	15%
Neurology	12–15%
Urology	7%
Thoracic	3–4%
General	2%
Orthopedic	1%
Oncology	Experimental
Dental	Experimental
Cardiovascular	Experimental

Figure 10. Surgical lasers: maturity of clinical applications.
Source: "Surgical Lasers: Market, Applications, and Trends," *Biomedical Business International* 10:12 (14 July 1978), 114.

clearly cannot rely on these programs for systematic and sustained technological growth. As the case of laser research demonstrates, defense spending can obstruct the evolution and the development of civilian technologies. Nevertheless, government efforts can facilitate collaboration among universities, firms, and government scientists to produce technologies desired by the government.

ENCOURAGING TECHNOLOGY TRANSFER

As we have seen, federal policies influenced the relationships among institutions in the research community. The dominance of NIH investigator-initiated grants solidified the strong connection between universities and the NIH. Significant research also occurred within the NIH in conjunction with its intramural research program. Innovative work often languished in universities and government laboratories without transfer to the private sector for commercialization.

Figure 11 captures these institutional barriers to the transfer of technology in the area of biomedical research. The link between the NIH and universities was very strong; the links between universities and government laboratories and the private sector were weak. Consequently, many innovative ideas were developed in academic and government laboratories, but they were never commercialized. This section explores the reasons for these problems and describes the public policies that were designed to help move technology along the innovation continuum.

University-Firm Relationships

In the early twentieth century, university researchers and industrial firms had little in common. Industrial research was not organized, and industrialists generally believed that the role of manufacturers was to make products. Contacts between firms and universities generally only occurred when university graduates entered firms as employees. Studies of the pharmaceutical industry between the wars revealed that researchers based in universities tended to denigrate the atmosphere in industry, which did not place a high value on research. As firms saw the benefits of research on the bottom line, however, they initiated modest interaction with universities.

In the 1940s and the early 1950s, contact between these two sectors was strengthened through fellowships, scholarships, and direct grants in aid from industry to institutions of higher learning. Individual consulting relationships developed between professors and firms. In that period, 300 firms engaged in forms of university support; 50 of them subsidized 270 biomedical projects at 70 different universities.[45]

Federal funding for scientific investigators burgeoned after

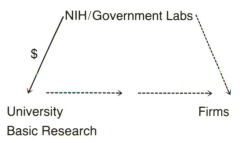

Figure 11. Institutional relationships in biomedical research.

World War II. The presence of federal money for biomedical research decreased incentives for individuals in universities to work with industry. It was much easier to go hat in hand to the NIH for support. Business-academic interactions reached their nadir in 1970, reflecting the high and consistent level in NIH support at the time. Academic institutions have typically received little direct payment from companies to which technology was transferred; most of the benefits have been indirect. The transfer has not generally occurred through licenses, but only when university trained students seek jobs in firms, when firms review academic journals, when individual professors are hired as consultants, or when researchers set up their own companies.[46]

Indeed, the general trend before 1980 was that most commercial technological advances did not pass through either government or university patent offices. Some start-up companies did negotiate licenses with the institutions where the founders had worked; others did not.

Universities had little incentive to push for patent rights. This lack of incentive is tied to government policy. Under the terms of federal grants, the federal agencies that paid for the research held the patents. Indeed, few universities even had formal patent or licensing offices; many had contract relationships with off-campus patent agents.[47] Many researchers failed to disclose their research because they either did not want to share revenue with the university or did not want to bother with the headaches of dealing with off-campus agents.

Because the NIH supported so much basic research, few researchers could claim patent rights in any case. The federal agencies were allowed to assign rights to the universities or to individual researchers, but intensive negotiation was required and rarely undertaken. Only institutions with extremely active research units bothered to establish patent offices. A study of the field of diagnostic imaging showed that institutions with patent offices tended to have more academic imaging products licensed.[48] Institutions with no patent office had few licenses even when the researchers were actively contributing to imaging innovation.[49]

By the late 1970s, shifts in government policy triggered changes in these institutional arrangements. The federal government began to reduce its commitment to federal research support. These cuts in federal biomedical research funding were exacerbated by the impact of inflation on research costs. Universities responded by encouraging contact with private industry, a potential source of research funds. One index of interaction is the flow of resources from firms to universities. The National Science Foundation estimated that corporate expenditures on university research would reach $670 million in 1987, up from $235 million in 1980.[50]

Corporate funds generally fall into three categories: gifts, research awards, and awards for instruction, equipment, and facilities. In fiscal year 1988 at the University of Michigan, for example, industry provided $104 million in gifts and grants (15.3 percent of total gift income) and $20.5 million in contract research expenditures (8.7 percent of total research expenditures). Research funds from industry rose 82 percent between 1983 and 1988, paralleling the growth in total university research expenditures. These figures do not include individual consulting relationships between faculty researchers and firms.[51]

Universities also developed significant formal institutional relationships with business, such as the creation of research parks and research consortia on or near campuses. Nearly four dozen universities have or are seriously considering the establishment of research parks, including Stanford, North Carolina, Duke, Yale, and Wisconsin. By 1988, Johns Hopkins University Medical School had over two hundred separate agreements with industry.[52]

Congress also initiated some affirmative policy changes. In 1980, it passed the Bayh-Dole Patent and Trademark Amendments.[53] This law gave nonprofit organizations, notably universities, rights to inventions made under federal grants and contracts. The new policy led to increased efforts by universities to report, license, and develop inventions. In 1984, the policy was extended to federal laboratories operated by universities and nonprofit corporations.[54] Many academic institutions have responded by creating patent, licensing, and industry liaison offices or by increasing the activity of existing offices. In 1985, for example, the total royalty income received by Stanford, MIT, and the University of California had risen from less than $5 million per year during the early 1980s to about $12.5 million annually. University of California revenue grew from $3.4 million to $5.4 million between 1985 and 1987 alone.[55]

Holding a patent will encourage technology transfer because licensing patent rights can be profitable. Universities have worked out elaborate policies for royalty sharing. Individual professors and the universities themselves stand to profit handsomely. The act of licensing transfers these innovative ideas to the private sector, a transfer that is consistent with the promotion of private sector initiatives and the downplaying of federal agencies that characterize the 1980s. Unlike the targeting approach of the 1970s, whereby a federal agency like the NIH decided what technologies to procure and paid for them to be developed, this new technology policy provides financial incentives in the private sector to promote technology transfer. The early data indicate that the incentives are working and that relationships between firms and universities have strengthened as a result.

Business-Government Relationships

Basic research also occurs in federal laboratories. The federal government spent approximately $18 billion in 1986 on research and development at over seven hundred federal laboratories. Although the NIH devotes only about 10 percent of its funds for in-house or intramural research, the research productivity of NIH scientists has grown steadily. Despite the fact that government laboratories have produced over 28,000 patents, only 5 percent have ever been licensed. Indeed, the NIH held few patents and practically gave away licenses. After all, the government scientists worked for salaries and were committed to research; the NIH had ample funds from Congress without supplementing income with licensing arrangements.

In 1980, Congress enacted the Stevenson-Wydler Technology Innovation Act to encourage the transfer of federal technology to industry.[56] Technology transfer from federal laboratories to industry became a national policy. The law created government offices to evaluate new technologies and to promote transfer, but it was not fully implemented or funded. Many of the federal laboratories lacked clear legal authority to enter into cooperative research projects.

In 1986, Congress passed the Federal Technology Transfer Act, amending Stevenson-Wydler to allow federal laboratories to enter into cooperative research with private industry, universities, and others.[57] It established a dual employee award system of sharing royalties between the agency and the individual researcher and making cash awards as well. Specifically, it provided for at least a 15 percent royalty payment to laboratory employees from the income received by the agency from the licensing of an invention. It also established a Consortium for Technology Transfer.

President Reagan issued an executive order in 1987 that called for enforcement and compliance with the law.[58] This order required that federal agencies "identify and encourage persons to act as conduits between and among federal laboratories, universities and the private sector for the transfer of technology, and to implement, as expeditiously as practicable, royalty sharing programs with inventors who were employees of the agency at the time their inventions were made, and cash award programs." Federal agencies in general, and the NIH in particular, struggled to define the parameters of relationships between its own scientists and commercial organizations. The NIH Office of Invention Development reported in 1989 that it reviewed four to five cooperative research and development agreements (CREDAS) each month.

Federal policies clearly have promoted innovation in biomedical sciences. How well have medical devices fared under these policies? The relationship between NIH and universities for promotion of basic scientific research benefits all scientific progress, which includes medical devices along with other medical technologies. However, the traditional bias of the NIH against engineering and other physical sciences has undoubtedly meant that some device technologies were overlooked. Most complex devices, particularly implantables, require a multidisciplinary approach to innovation. An unduly narrow focus on biochemistry and pharmacology at the expense of physics, engineering, and biomaterials science would not promote development in those fields.

The medical device industry stands to benefit from policy changes that have promoted government links with private industry. Congressional efforts to direct the NIH toward targeted development have supported some medical device innovation. The support provided to small innovators pursuing long-term investigations undoubtedly has fostered technology that would otherwise be abandoned. The Artificial Heart Program illustrates both the strengths and the weaknesses of the approach. Clearly, some innovative firms, and some technology, would not exist without NIH support.

Similarly, the recent efforts to strengthen the relationship of universities and government labs to private firms will also benefit the device industry. As with targeted development, this approach erodes the traditional focus on basic science, emphasizing instead the commercial potential of new ideas. Collaboration with universities presents positive opportunities for the device industry. Because of the multidisciplinary nature of device development, the more alternative routes available to an innovator the better.

These changes raise significant social issues that are often overlooked. Is government targeting of medical technology a wise use of public funds? Are these products different from other goods, justifying public expenditures for product development? Such a view "assumes that if a potential capability exists to cure a life-threatening disease, there exists a moral obligation to develop that capability. It is a kind of extension of the philosophy underlying the Hippocratic oath to the development of new technologies."[59]

Other issues arise when taxpayers' money is used to develop products. Should these beneficial products be turned over to the private firms who will make a profit on them? What if the products developed with government funds are so expensive that some citizens will not be able to afford them? The artificial heart will be an extraordinarily expensive technology. Does it make any difference whether the source of funds was public or private or whether the product is widely available? Is it equally immoral for government to fail to promote a lifesaving or life-enhancing technology if there is the basic knowledge to develop it but no source of private funds?

How well does government pick technologies to promote? There is contentious debate over the wisdom of industrial policy, which refers to deliberate government programs that channel resources to particular industrial sectors to promote or protect them. Does government have the skill to pick winners in the medical marketplace?

Additional issues arise in relation to the institutional changes discussed above. Some have called the federal policies to strengthen the ties of university and government laboratories to industry misguided because of the institutional effects. They ask, for example, whether the profit motive will subvert the scientific missions of universities and government researchers, who may be lured by profits from the private sector and ignore the pursuit of knowledge for its own sake. Will conflicts of interest between public employees and the private sector arise as a result? Some fear that the NIH will become a private procurement lab for industry. Who will engage in the long-term scientific investigations with no immediate commercial potential if professors are busy collaborating with industry? Will academic researchers hesitate to disclose their findings until the patents are filed, thereby restricting the free flow of information at scientific meetings? Secrecy is antithetical to scientific progress, but it is essential to profitmaking in a competitive environment.

These tantalizing questions are not easy to answer. However, they illustrate the complex issues raised by government promotion of medical discoveries, questions we will explore further in the concluding chapter. Now we turn to government promotion of medical device distribution—the other end of the innovation continuum.

4

GOVERNMENT PROMOTES
MEDICAL DEVICE DISTRIBUTION

	Discovery	Distribution
Promote	1. National Institutes of Health (NIH) Space & Defense Spinoffs	2. Hill-Burton Hospital Construction Funds Medicare/Medicaid
Inhibit	3. Regulation (FDA) Product Liability	4. Certificate of Need Cost-Containment Technology Assessment

Figure 12. The policy matrix.

Throughout the 1950s and 1960s, the federal government remained firmly committed to promoting biomedical research. Public belief in the benefits of technology characterized this period. As technological improvements in medical treatment emerged after World War II, many people were priced out of the increasingly sophisticated and desirable medical market. At the same time, there was growing belief that it was immoral not to provide some level of health care to everyone who needed it.

Demand for access to health care increased. The economics of health soon became a political issue. In a variety of ways, government accepted greater social responsibility for the structure of health care delivery and access for excluded groups. Indeed, the public sector moved from a refusal to become involved in health care to the nation's largest single purchaser of services in a relatively brief period. By the mid-1980s, public funds accounted for 20 percent of health care spending and 40 percent of payments to hospitals.[1]

This chapter examines how the government commitment to health care has influenced the medical device industry from the postwar period until 1983. Our examination breaks at that juncture because massive changes in the structure of the federal payment system that year ushered in the era of cost containment. In the period before 1983, government policy promoted distribution of medical device technology. The entry of government led to unrestrained growth in the demand for medical devices. Government policy encouraged acquisition regardless of cost and was biased toward growth of hospital based technology. Government affected both the size and the composition of the medical device market. (See figure 12.)

As a third-party payer, rather than a provider of services, government refrained from direct involvement in treatment decisions. The result was only tenuous control over total program costs. These policies provide the background for the cost-containment efforts of the late 1970s and 1980s that will be discussed in chapter 7.

This chapter illustrates the impact of government policy through three case studies. The story of the artificial kidney shows how government spending literally created the market for this expensive, lifesaving technology. The introduction of the CT scanner, a computer assisted X-ray device that revolutionized diagnostic imaging, illustrates the effect of government spending policy on the diffusion of high-cost capital equipment. Finally, the rapid growth of the cardiac pacemaker market reveals how unrestrained payment can lead to market abuse.

A brief caveat before proceeding: Medicare and Medicaid are extremely complex public policies, and the discussion here is inevitably cursory. This chapter examines the impact of the government payment systems on medical devices. Many less pertinent, but otherwise important, aspects of these payment schemes are not discussed. Interested readers should consult the notes for more detailed studies.

POLICY OVERVIEW, 1950–1983

Hill-Burton Promotes Hospital Growth

Very little hospital construction took place during the depression and World War II. After the war, however, there was both a general belief that hospital beds were in short supply and much concern about the uneven distribution of beds among the states and between rural and urban areas.[2] Congress passed the Hospital Survey and Construction Act of 1946, which has come to be known as Hill-Burton, the names of its congressional sponsors.[3] Hill-Burton represented an unprecedented involvement of the federal government in facilitating access to health care. The objectives of the new legislation were to survey the need for construction and to aid in the building of public and other nonprofit hospitals.

Consistent with ongoing concerns about the propriety of federal involvement in health services, the program was set up as a federal and state partnership. An agency in each state was designated as the state approved Hill-Burton organization and was given an initial grant to survey hospital needs. The state then received funds to carry out the construction program, subject to federal approval. Priority was given to states where shortages were the greatest. The ultimate allotment formula was based on the state's relative population and its per capita income. The poorer and the more rural the state, the greater the level of federal funds available to it.

In the period of 1946–1971, short-term acute or general hospitals received the largest share of Hill-Burton support, averaging over 71 percent of program funds. While Hill-Burton funds did not dominate spending on hospital facilities, their impact on hospitals was high. Between 1949 and 1962, the federal government paid directly about 10 percent of the annual costs of all hospital construction under the program. In other words, about 30 percent of all hospital construction projects received some form of federal assistance.[4]

The number of available hospital beds grew accordingly. In 1948, there were 469,398 short-term beds; by 1969, the number had almost doubled to 826,711. Of these, 40 percent had been partially supported by Hill-Burton monies.[5] Studies indicate that the program had a generally significant effect on the change in hospital beds per capita between 1947 and 1970.[6] In particular, it increased the number of hospital beds in smaller cities and targeted low-income states.

The impact clearly favored the growth of short-term acute care facilities. Some years after the program began, there was a recognition of the bias in favor of these institutions. In 1954, Congress amended the law to provide grants to assist with out-patient facilities and long-term care facilities. In 1964, additional changes earmarked funds specifically for modernization of older facilities rather than for a further increase of beds. Despite these amendments, the thrust of the program was expansion of acute care facilities. Government funds essentially established the mix of facilities in the marketplace. The result was growth of the potential market for medical technology appropriately designed for these settings. The beds were available; the problem then became access to this costly and sophisticated hospital care.

The Pressure for Access Grows

Expansion of hospitals inevitably led to pressure to provide more services as hospitals sought to fill their beds. During the prewar period, particularly during the depression, families denied themselves medical care. However, medicine now offered more benefits than ever before, particularly in the modern hospital setting. In response, interest groups began to press for policies that would increase access to these new and expensive therapies. Some turned to government as the logical source of funds for health care services. However, reformers confronted the traditional long-standing objection to federal involvement in health care services.

This opposition to federal entry into health care was intense. In stark contrast to the expansion of Social Security during the postwar period, there was a political deadlock over state supported health insurance proposals.[7] Physicians, represented by the American Medical Association (AMA), and many business groups strongly opposed all forms of national health insurance.

The AMA denounced disability insurance as "another step toward wholesale nationalization of medical care and the socialization of the practice of medicine."[8]

The debate has been characterized as partly ideological, partly social, and partly material. For all these reasons, compulsory national health insurance was not forthcoming in the 1950s. Only American veterans received extensive, federally supported medical care through Veterans Administration hospitals that were greatly expanded during the postwar period. "The AMA opposed the extension of the veterans' program to nonservice connected illness, but the veterans were one lobby even the medical profession could not overcome."[9] There is real irony in this physician-led opposition to federal health programs given both the subsequent expansion of the patient base through Medicare and Medicaid and the flow of millions of dollars to physicians from government coffers.

Although the government remained intransigent, there were options in the private sector for some groups. The middle class continued to seek forms of private insurance coverage; unions began to look for health benefits in collective bargaining agreements. By the 1950s, there was a stable pattern of growth in private insurance coverage, expanding the market for health care to the employed and the middle class. Much of the insurance was available to working people as fringe benefits; labor managed to bargain successfully for health insurance. By mid-1958, nearly two-thirds of the population had some insurance coverage for hospital costs. The higher the family income, the more likely that it had insurance. In 1948, 72 percent of patients paid directly for health care and only 6 percent had any form of private third-party insurance. By 1966, 52 percent of patients paid directly for health care and 25 percent had private insurance (see table 2). The numbers that received care from public funds remained relatively stable—19 percent in 1948 and only 21 percent by 1966. The poor received welfare and charity care when they could. The retired, unemployed, and disabled were often virtually excluded from the benefits of hospital based care.

The availability of insurance provided stability to the market and increased market size. The financing mechanisms through

Table 2. Sources of Payment for Personal Health Care Expenditures

	Private patient	*Third-party payment*	
	---	---	---
Year	*Direct payment*	*Private insurers*	*Public funds*
1948	72%	6%	19%
1966	52%	25%	21%
1982	25%	32%	41%

Sources: U.S. Department of Commerce, Bureau of the Census, *Statistical Abstract of the United States: 1985,* Table 143 (Washington, D.C., 1984); *Historical Statistics of the United States: Colonial Times to 1970*, Series B, 242–247 (Washington, D.C., 1975). Reprinted from Susan Bartlett Foote, "From Crutches to CT Scans: Business-Government Relations and Medical Product Innovation," *Research in Corporate Social Performance and Policy* 8 (1986), 3–28.

Numbers do not sum to 100%. Balance is "other" private payment.

payroll withholding kept spending stable during recessions and reduced market uncertainty for providers and suppliers. Although causality is difficult to document, the growth in private health care expenditures during this period did expand the market for medical products, particularly in the hospital sector. The value of medical product shipments, based on data in the SIC codes, began to climb, and sales in the five relevant SIC categories rose at an average annual rate of 6 percent, which is three times the growth rate immediately before World War II but less than half of the wartime rate of increase.[10] Table 3 captures the boom in sales during this period.

Despite the growth of private insurance, pressure to expand access to health care from those outside the medical care system continued. Some favored a compulsory and contributory health insurance system. Although legislation had been introduced as early as 1958, the real impetus came after the Democratic sweep of the presidency and the Congress in 1964. In 1965, President Johnson signed the Medicare Amendments to the Social Security Act in which the federal government definitively entered the marketplace. The new law's intention was to open the health care system to the elderly. The president declared: "Every citizen will be able, in his productive years when he is earning, to insure

Table 3. Real (1972) Dollar Value of Shipments of Medical Devices, by SIC Code, Selected Years, 1958–1983 (in millions of dollars)

Year	X-ray and electromedical equipment (SIC 3693)	Surgical and medical instruments (SIC 3841)	Surgical appliances and supplies (SIC 3842)	Dental equipment and supplies (SIC 3843)	Ophthalmic goods (SIC 3851)	Total
1983[a]	$2,145	$2,050	$2,975	$540	NA	$7,710[b]
1982	1,858	1,915	2,790	528	$757	7,848
1981	1,374	1,587	2,337	659	704	6,661
1980	1,210	1,494	2,007	685	735	6,131
1977	1,274	1,273	1,649	564	707	5,467
1972	444	962	1,454	409	568	3,837
1967	311	568	920	234	479	2,512
1963	217	377	705	160	312	1,771
1958	150	184	549	130	231	1,244

Source: Federal Policies and the Medical Devices Industry (Washington, D.C.: Office of Technology Assessment, 19 October 1984), 19.

[a] Estimates.

[b] Total does not include shipments of ophthalmic goods.

himself against the ravages of illness in his old age. . . . No longer will illness crush and destroy the savings that they have so carefully put away over a lifetime."[11]

Medicare in Brief

This section briefly examines the key attributes of the Medicare insurance program through 1983, at which time occurred a massive restructuring to contain costs.[12] Medicare's hospital insurance program, Part A, covered specific hospital inpatient services for the elderly and some other extended care. Part B, Medicare's supplementary medical insurance program, covered costs associated with physicians and hospital outpatient services and various other kinds of limited ambulatory care. Part A is supported by the Medicare trust fund and is available to all elderly citizens. Part B is a voluntary program, supported by subscriber payments and congressional appropriations. In 1972, Medicare eligibility was extended to disabled persons and most persons with end-stage renal disease (ESRD), those with kidney failure (see table 4).[13]

Moreover, the Medicare-eligible population has greater health needs than the average citizen. While the elderly constitute about 11.2 percent of the population, they account for 31.4 percent of the health care costs.[14] By the mid-1980s, Medicare became the largest single payer for hospital services, accounting for 28 percent of the nation's hospital bills. Medicare also accounted for a significant portion of funds for physician payments under Part B.[15]

The Medicare program had an immediate and significant impact on medical devices. Medicare costs are tied to the dollars paid by the government for services provided under the programs. The method of reimbursement was a cost-plus system that retroactively compensated providers for all "necessary and proper" expenses associated with treatment for the covered individuals. This system encouraged the purchase and use of medical technology.

Reimbursement rates for Medicare patients included a capital cost pass-through, which meant that hospitals could receive reimbursement for capital expenditures to the extent that those

Table 4. Number of Elderly and Disabled Beneficiaries Enrolled in Medicare by Type of Coverage, Selected Years from 1966 to 1982

Enrollment year[a]	Total number of Medicare beneficiaries	Number of elderly[b] beneficiaries	Number of disabled[c] beneficiaries	Number of elderly and disabled beneficiaries with ESRD
1966	19,108,822	19,108,822	—	—
1973	23,545,363	21,814,825	1,730,538	NA
1974	24,201,042	22,272,920	1,928,122	18,564
1979	27,858,742	24,947,954	2,910,788	60,608
1982	29,494,219	26,539,994	2,954,225	76,117

Source: Department of Health and Human Services, Health Care Financing Administration, *1966–1979 Data Notes: Persons Enrolled for Medicare, 1979*, HCFA publication no. 03079 (Baltimore, Md.: HCFA, January 1981); and H. A. Silverman, Medicare Program Statistics Branch, HCFA, personal communication, August 1983. Reprinted from *Medical Technology and Costs of the Medicare Program* (Washington, D.C.: Office of Technology Assessment, July 1984), 27.

[a]Enrollment year begins July 1.

[b]All beneficiaries aged 65 and over, including those with end-stage renal disease.

[c]All beneficiaries under age 65, including those with end-stage renal disease.

capital costs were part of Medicare services. (Capital expenditures generally include durable medical equipment, such as beds, operating room machinery, and diagnostic equipment.) Hospital administrators had little reason to resist pressure from physicians and others to buy new, specialized, and perhaps underutilized equipment. Indeed, the growing prevalence of third-party financing, particularly in the public sector, is considered one of the major causes of inflation in hospital costs.[16] Much of those costs were associated with spending on medical devices.

The Medicare system is administered by the Health Care Financing Administration (HCFA). The HCFA contracts with private organizations, such as Blue Cross and Blue Shield, to process the claims. Private insurers, called *fiscal intermediaries*, handle claims under Part A of the program; insurers for Part B are called *carriers*. Figure 13 illustrates the complicated process for Medicare claims.

Claims processing is an enormous undertaking. In 1987, HCFA processed approximately 366 million Medicare claims.[17] In addition, HCFA also handles disputes about whether Medicare covers a particular procedure or technology. To be eligible for Medicare payment, there must be a determination that a new technology or device will be covered. Indeed, advisors to the Department of Health and Human Services concluded in a recent report that "Medicare coverage policy involves so large a portion of U.S. health care delivery that it can significantly affect the diffusion of a technology as well as the environment for technological innovation."[18]

The Medicare Act prohibited payment for any items or service not considered reasonable and necessary for patient care. However, the law did not include a comprehensive list of items or services considered "reasonable and necessary" under the program. Medicare coverage policy continuously evolved and was implemented in a decentralized manner. Some coverage decisions were made at a national level by HCFA's central office, under advice from the federal Office of Health Technology Assessment (OHTA).[19] Most decisions were made by Medicare contractors who processed claims. The decentralized nature of the process can create an uncertain marketplace for newly introduced technologies. However, in the early years of the federal program, coverage decisions were consistently favorable for devices and the complex process was little threat to the industry.

Medicaid in Brief

The 1965 law also established the Medicaid program, a silent partner to Medicare that received much more publicity at the time. The goals and structure of Medicaid are quite different than Medicare. Its purpose is to provide payment for medical care for certain low-income families defined by law as medically needy. The goal is to increase access of the poor to health care services.[20]

Unlike Medicare, which is a wholly federal program, Medicaid uses a combination of federal and state funds but states

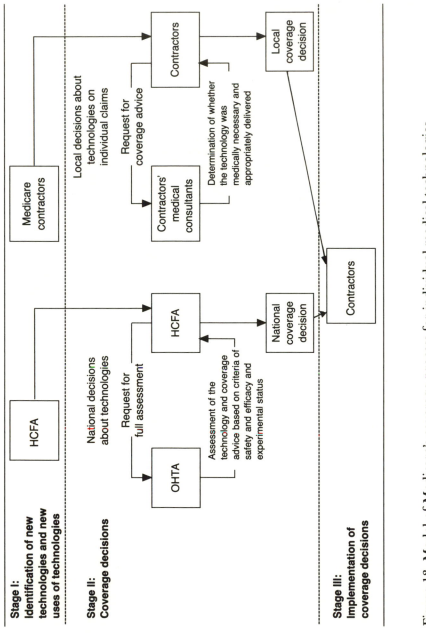

Figure 13. Model of Medicare's coverage process for individual medical technologies.
Source: Medical Technology and Costs of the Medicare Program (Washington, D.C.: Office of Technology Assessment, July 1984), 76.

control and administer them. Medicare is tied to Social Security and has uniform national standards for eligibility and benefits. Medicaid, however, defers to the states on many aspects of its programs for the poor and places more restrictions on physician participation. States are not required to participate in Medicaid, but elaborate financial incentives virtually guarantee participation. By 1977, all states had a Medicaid program in place. States may impose complicated eligibility requirements and benefits vary significantly from state to state. States set the definition of income limits for an individual or a family. These limits differ considerably among the states. Many families below the federally defined poverty line are not eligible for Medicaid in some states.[21]

The federal government matches the state expenditures in the program based on a formula tied to each state's per capita income. The federal contribution to the program ranges from approximately 50 to 78 percent of the state's total costs.[22] When Medicaid was passed, supporters argued that it would add only $250 million to the health care expenditures of the federal government. In the first year of the program, the outlays of the federal and state governments were $1.5 billion. By 1975, spending rose to $14.2 billion, and in 1987 the expenditures exceeded $47 billion (see figure 14).

The number of people enrolled in the programs has increased as well. There were 4.5 million recipients in 1968 and 24 million in 1977, at Medicaid's peak; the figure dropped to 23.2 million in 1987. Medicaid accounted for over 10 percent of America's total health care expenses in the 1980s. At that time the distribution of recipients included dependent children under twenty-one years of age, adults in families with dependent children, persons over sixty-five, the permanently and totally disabled, and the blind. The types of services covered include inpatient, acute care, skilled nursing homes, mental hospitals, physicians services, and outpatient and clinic services. However, inpatient services (including hospitals and nursing homes) constitute about 70 percent of Medicaid payments.[23]

The program has been tremendously controversial. It has been criticized for rapidly rising costs, well-documented claims of fraud and abuse by providers, and questions about manage-

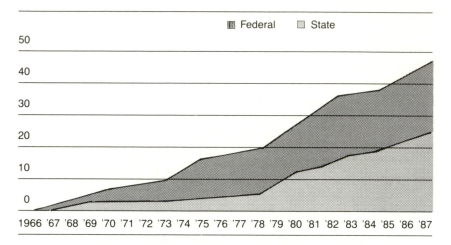

Figure 14. Federal and state Medicaid expenditures, 1966–1987 (in billions of dollars).

Source: Health Care Financing Administration. Reprinted from Oberg and Polichj, "Medicaid: Entering the Third Decade," *Health Affairs* (Fall 1988), 85.

ment, quality, and equity. But Medicaid remains the primary vehicle for access to health care for the nation's poor.

Impact on Medical Device Sales

These two major health initiatives led to greatly increased spending on health. National health care expenditures rose from $40.46 billion in 1965, which was 5.9 percent of the GNP, to $322.3 billion, or 10.5 percent of the GNP, by 1982. Per capita expenditures increased more than fivefold, from $207 in 1965 to $1,337 in 1982. The public share of coverage rose from only 21 percent in 1966 to 41 percent in 1982.

It is clear that private insurance programs helped to increase and to stabilize the health care market generally. However, the infusion of capital from federal and state governments brought millions of heretofore excluded individuals into the system.

Without question, government spending significantly expanded the marketplace for health care services and, inevitably, for medical devices associated with treatment. In general, hospitals benefited the most by federal and state spending programs, but device sales increased in all relevant categories. Examination of the individual SIC categories of medical devices supports the conclusion that federal spending expanded industry sales. In 1982, hospitals purchased $7 billion of the $16.8 billion in sales of products in the five SIC codes, and this total does not include some infrequently purchased larger items (see table 5).

Three SIC categories—3693: X-ray, electromedical, and electrotherapeutic apparatus; 3841: surgical and medical supplies; and 3842: surgical appliances and supplies—are particularly closely tied to federal Medicare and Medicaid payments because of their strong association with a hospital base. Dental and ophthalmic supplies (SIC 3843 and 3851 respectively) are less likely to be covered by Medicare payments. Before Medicare, four of the five SIC categories had similar growth patterns from 1945 to 1965; the fifth, surgical and medical instruments, grew faster because of demand stimulated by hospital construction. After 1965, however, sales in the three Medicare affected categories were much higher (14 to 22 percent) than the other two (8 to 11 percent).[24]

The following case studies illustrate more specifically the powerful impact of federal spending on medical device growth.

GOVERNMENT POLICY AND MEDICAL DEVICE DISTRIBUTION

Government programs dominated segments of the medical device market and had an enormous impact on the size and composition of those market segments. Government policies for payment can create or eliminate a product market or can force the product to move from one market segment to another. As the leading force in paying for medical services, the government indirectly shaped the market for medical device innovations.

Government Influences Market Size: The Case of Kidney Dialysis

The kidneys maintain the equilibrium of dozens of chemicals in the body, control the pressure, acidity, and volume of blood, and filter the blood to remove excess fluid and waste products.

Table 5. Sales of Selected Medical Devices to Hospitals by
SIC Code, 1982
(in thousands of dollars)

SIC code/product	Sales to hospitals
X-ray and electromedical equipment (SIC 3693)	
X-ray supplies	$ 777,366
Radiological catheters and guide wire	135,878
Pacemakers and other cardiovascular products	499,999
Electrosurgical supplies	48,552
Surgical and medical instruments (SIC 3841)	
Surgeons' needles	4,310
Blood collection supplies	57,845
Thermometers	31,426
Surgical instruments	294,284
Syringes and needles	331,054
Catheters, tubes, and allied products	235,445
Diagnostic instruments	69,549
Surgical appliances and supplies (SIC 3842)	
Sutures	286,635
Ostomy products	13,842
Surgical packs and parts	174,123
Maternity products	26,869
Dialysis supplies	97,677
Cardiopulmonary supplies	71,176
Sponges	174,768
Bandages, dressings, and elastic	172,303
Orthopedic supplies	302,283
Parenteral supplies	701,106
Urological products	198,970
Sterilizer supplies	88,846
Cast room supplies	39,836
Disposable kits and trays	258,317
Respiratory therapy	245,890
Garments, textiles, and gloves	592,254
Ophthalmic goods (SIC 3851)	
Ophthalmic related products	83,649
Other	
Solutions	872,985

Table 5. *continued*

SIC code/product	Sales to hospitals
Other (continued)	
Medical supplies	420,702
Chemicals and soaps	153,946
Paper products	113,738
Gases	109,933
Underpads	55,259
Identification supplies	31,517
Elastic goods	24,932
Rubber goods	7,281
Total	$7,804,545

Source: IMS America, Ltd. Rockville, Md., unpublished data, 1983. Reprinted from *Federal Policies and the Medical Devices Industry* (Washington, D.C.: Office of Technology Assessment, October 1984), 24.

Kidneys can be damaged by diseases, infections, obstructions, toxins, or shock, any of which can lead to end-stage renal disease (ESRD). When the kidneys fail, the body swells with water and accumulates wastes and poisons. The individual may become comatose and may ultimately die.

Hemodialysis is the term used to describe the kidney's filtration of blood. The artificial kidney accomplishes hemodialysis through diffusion, which rids the body of toxins, and ultrafiltration, which removes excess fluid.[25] The developmental history of hemodialysis dates back to the early 1900s. Early experiments confirmed the conceptual basis for dialysis, but there remained several barriers—particularly the lack of anticoagulants and an effective filtration membrane. The development of compound heparin solved the first problem; commercial production of cellophane solved the second.[26]

Willem J. Kolff developed the first artificial kidney machine in Holland in the 1940s. The first American machine was built in 1947, in collaboration with researchers at Peter Bent Brigham Hospital. This equipment worked well on patients suffering acute kidney failure. However, patients with chronic kidney failure could survive only if they remained connected to the machine. The problem was that of access to the veins; each connection required surgical operations. With the invention of the Quinton-Scribner shunt in 1959, a device that permitted repeated connections, the machine could be used for patients with chronic kidney failure. It is interesting to note that the critical material in the shunt was Teflon, an inert fluorocarbon resin that the body did not reject.[27]

By the early 1960s, patients were receiving dialysis experimentally in Seattle, and the country began to be aware of this new lifesaving technology. Hemodialysis costs were high because of the hospital space required, the expensive machinery, and the need for trained personnel. In 1967, for example, the Veterans Administration Hospital in Los Angeles estimated the cost of dialysis at $28,000 per year per patient. Because of these high costs, the number of people receiving dialysis in the 1960s remained small. There were approximately 800 dialysis patients in 121 centers in 1967, many of whom were subsidized by funds from voluntary agencies.[28] The small size of the dialysis market operated as a disincentive to innovation and production.

> There were always equipment vendors ready to sell artificial kidneys to prospective buyers, even prior to the Quinton-Scribner shunt. The scarce resource was never machines, but money. But the few companies that did supply both machines and disposables for dialysis supported very little R&D directed to developing a better artificial kidney. Unit costs for kidney machines were high, the buyers were few, and the financial means for paying for treatment costs for the potential patient pool were uncertain in all but a few cases. There were simply no market incentives for private investment in R&D in building better artificial kidneys.[29]

Access to the limited number of kidney dialysis units became a highly charged public issue. Patients turned away from the treatment would die within weeks. Centers began to create priorities for patients, sometimes based on concepts of the relative social worth of individuals. Government policy in the past had approached medical problems through disease specific interventions (such as the Heart Disease, Cancer, and Stroke Act), but the dominant policy was to support basic research and evaluate the products of research.[30] The delivery of services was left to the private market, except in the cases of the elderly under Medicare and the indigent under Medicaid. For kidney failure, there was an available technology that worked. The problem for patients was how to pay for it.

Congress responded in 1972 by amending the Social Security Act. The new law provided federal reimbursement for nearly all the costs of dialysis for virtually every person with ESRD. The impact was immediate. Government policy dramatically increased the size of the market for dialysis equipment and supplies. In 1972, forty patients per million in population were receiving long-term dialysis in the United States, primarily supported by nonprofit organizations.[31] By 1977 there were 895 approved facilities, providing 7,306 dialysis stations and serving over 27,000 patients. By 1980 there were 50,000 long-term hemodialysis patients; by 1982 there were 58,391.

In addition to increasing the number of patients, the federal policies favored hospital based or community based dialysis over home dialysis. Nearly 40 percent of the patients were being dialyzed in their homes at the time of the 1972 law. The percentage declined significantly, to about 13 percent, by 1980. The shift to the costlier treatment centers occurred because home dialysis was reimbursed under Part B of Medicare, which meant that fewer items were covered than in hospital and community dialysis centers under Part A. There were, of course, other relevant factors in addition to reimbursement, including the stress on family life of home dialysis and the increased age and morbidity of dialysis patients as the treatment became more common. Despite subsequent amendments to realign the incentives to encourage home dialysis, the costs of the ESRD program mounted. The actual costs of the program in 1974 were $242.5 million. By 1983, the program cost Medicare $2.2 billion.[32]

It is clear that the dialysis equipment industry thrived in this growing, publicly financed marketplace. Indeed, it has been said that "governmental intervention in the marketplace has been the single most important factor influencing both supply and demand" for the ESRD related equipment industry.[33] Within five years of the establishment of the ESRD program, yearly sales in the dialysis industry were nearly $300 million.

The renal dialysis equipment industry includes firms that

manufacture and distribute dialyzers or artificial kidneys, delivery and monitoring equipment, and disposable equipment such as blood tubing, connectors, and needles and syringes.[34] The industry is highly concentrated, with the three largest firms sharing 72.1 percent of the kidney machine marketplace in the mid-1970s. Suppliers of hemodialysis related products were slightly less concentrated. Baxter Travenol was the clear industry leader, with 40 percent of the total market by the mid-1970s. Its sales and earnings records were outstanding during the 1960s and 1970s, with "ongoing market expansion and new kidney dialysis products" as a key to the firm's success.[35]

Baxter flourished in an environment where price competition was rather limited. The role of government as the primary payer has been found to intensify nonprice competition. The prosperity of the industry was linked to federal dollars. By the late 1970s, large corporate firms such as Johnson & Johnson and Eli Lilly entered the ESRD market by acquiring smaller existing firms. Baxter continued to lead the field, with 38 percent of the disposable market and 34 percent of the equipment market in 1981.

There is controversy about the government's role in kidney dialysis, particularly in regard to the costs of the program. Indeed, ESRD patients represent only one-quarter of 1 percent of Medicare beneficiaries, but they consume about 4 percent of total Medicare benefit payments. There is concern that patients with poor prognoses are given treatment that cannot improve the quality of their lives. Some argue that perverse incentives in the payment structure have directed dialysis patients to more expensive centers rather than to lower-cost home dialysis. The debate illustrates the hard questions of allocation of medical resources. Advocates of universal dialysis say the United States can afford it; others question the wisdom of this expensive program, rejecting the accusation of lack of compassion for kidney patients.

I do not believe we can satisfy all the health care needs of our citizens. If that is the case, we cannot solve the problem by showing more compassion since compassionately providing care for some will require depriving others of the care they need. In this context, then, the question of how best to use our limited health care funds becomes crucially important.[36]

Government Influences Distribution: The Case of CT Scanners

The invention of the X-ray greatly enhanced physicians' ability to diagnose medical problems. Computed tomography (CT) represents a significant technological advance over earlier technologies that produce images to aid in diagnosis of disease.[37] CT scanners are more sensitive to variations in bone and tissue density than X-rays are, and they produce images with greater resolution and speed, thereby reducing the patient's exposure to radiation.

Computed tomography relies on X-ray images. However, CT emits X-rays from multiple sources, and multiple electronic receptors surrounding the patient receive them. The information from the multiple views is processed by a computer that reconstructs the "slice" of the patient's body. The CT scan has a superior ability to differentiate among soft tissues (such as the liver, spleen, or kidney) and provides a much better depiction of the anatomy and the diseases affecting these tissues than do previous technologies. Indeed, the range of density recorded increases from about 20 with conventional X-rays, or as little as 1 percent of the information in the ray, to more than 2,000 with CT scans.[38]

Radon, a German researcher, worked out the early mathematical basis for the reconstruction of images from projections in 1917. Research continued during the 1950s, and in 1961, neurologist William Oldendorf constructed a tomographic device at UCLA and received the first patent in 1962. Despite subsequent work, corporations and physicians showed no interest in commercial development.[39]

The first commercial interest in CT occurred in Britain. Godfrey Hounsfield, an engineer at the labs of EMI, a British electronics firm, developed a CT instrument in 1967. No X-ray companies wanted to license CT technology. However, the British Department of Health supported the construction of a prototype head scanner in the early 1970s. The Mayo Clinic installed the first X-ray scanner in the United States in June 1973.[40] By the end of the year, there were six EMI head scanners in the United States. Orders poured in following the showing of EMI's first-generation head scanner at the November 1973 meetings of the Radiological Society of North America. The price of the original scanners was about $400,000. There was widespread diffusion within four years, despite the high cost and the high annual operating expenses (approximately $400,000). During 1974, American sales were almost $20 million; in 1975, EMI shipped 120 units and reached sales of $60 million. The market continued to grow in the 1970s; corporate entry matched sales growth as competitors entered the American market.[41]

Technical improvements followed, and the units moved through four generations of operating methods within four years. The first generation was the EMI head scanner that used one X-ray generator to produce a single beam of radiation that was captured in one detector. By 1975 the second generation used two or more beams and two or more detectors, producing images significantly faster. In 1976 the third-generation head scanners used a single fan beam and hundreds of contiguous detectors. The NIH had become interested by this time and contracted with American Science and Engineering (AS&E) to develop a scanner. In 1976, AS&E introduced a commercial fourth-generation body scanner that produced images in under five seconds using a fan beam source and rotating detectors.

Numerous firms entered the fast-growing field. General Electric became the leading manufacturer with a market share of 60 percent by 1981.[42] It achieved success by acquiring the CT operations of several competitors, and its design dominated the CT market. Because of GE's reputation and size, buyers trusted that it would remain in business and shied away from new, potentially unstable companies.

By 1983 the CT market reached $750 million. The rate of adoption and the diffusion of this expensive piece of equipment was extremely rapid in its first ten years. Government money is not the only factor relevant to rapid diffusion. CT represented a major clinical breakthrough, and there were no real uncertainties during the first few years regarding the possible outdating of the core technology. For clinical reasons alone, acquisition made sense.

However, the price was very high. The availability of federal reimbursement dollars made the acquisition decision easier for hospitals. The diffusion of CT occurred entirely during the era of cost-based hospital reimbursement that promoted technology acquisition. Medicare had developed a complicated capital-cost pass-through program that permitted hospitals to submit capital-cost reports to Medicare to recoup a percentage of capital investments based on the share of Medicare participation in designated hospital departments. All operating costs of the technology were billed on the basis of the "reasonable and necessary" test.[43]

Although there were some efforts to control technology diffusion by the mid-1970s, most states did not have viable regulations affecting hospital acquisition at this time.[44] Where there was control on hospital purchasing, however, the response was an increase in the number of outpatient CT scanners. About 19 percent were placed outside the hospital in the first four years of availability overall, but outpatient siting was much higher in states such as New York and Massachusetts because they had some constraints in place.[45]

Many studies have compared CT diffusion with the subsequent introduction of magnetic resonance imaging (MRI), a newer, competitive imaging technology. MRI was introduced in the 1980s, when cost-containment policies were more mature.[46] The studies reveal that federal cost controls have played a major role in slowing diffusion rates for MRI. The conclusions underscore the theme that government payment policies in the 1960s and 1970s promoted widespread diffusion of medical technologies regardless of cost.

Government Policies and Fraud: The Case of Pacemakers

Given the incentive structure of the Medicare system, it is not surprising that there were abuses. The market for cardiac pacemakers, sold and implanted almost exclusively in elderly Medicare recipients, was rife with fraud. The technology itself is

lifesaving; it was unnecessary implantation and excessive competition in the industry that caused problems. The development
of the technology illustrates the best in creative innovation; the
subsequent misuse of the product represents the shameful side
of the medical technology market.

The adult heart beats as many as one hundred thousand times
a day. The steady beating is regulated by a natural pacemaker,
called the *sinus node,* which is located in the atrium, or upper
right chamber of the heart. An electrical impulse travels to the
bottom heart chambers, the ventricles, through a midway junction, the A-V node. This sequence causes the heart to contract. If
the electrical signals are sent too slowly, or if the junction is
blocked, the individual will experience shortness of breath, dizzi-
ness, fainting, convulsions, and death.

The concept of heart stimulation by external means dates
back to the 1800s. However, the development of a totally implantable device that could stimulate the regular beating of the
heart required the confluence of numerous technological advancements. Once these technologies were available, someone
had to have the vision to recognize the medical need and develop the product.[47]

The pacemaker depended on innovation in semiconductor
and electronics technology, principally the transistor, which became available in 1948. In addition, sophisticated battery technology was necessary for circuitry operation. World War II had
stimulated the development of improved sealed alkaline dry-cell
batteries that allowed the pacemaker system to be encapsulated
in a resin and implanted. The pacing system, which comes in
contact with cardiac tissue, required lead wires that were mechanically strong, relatively low-resistant, and well insulated
against leakage. Finally, the product required silicone rubber
and epoxy resins—biomaterials compatible with human tissue.

The market for such a heart-pacing device became apparent
to some physicians with the first open-heart surgery in the late
1950s. To stimulate the heart after surgery, physicians had used
bulky units that plugged into wall outlets and applied strong
currents to the patient's heart. Wilson Greatbatch, an electrical
engineer, began work on an implantable permanent cardiac
pacemaker in the mid-1950s while he was at the University of

Buffalo.[48] He found little interest in his pacemaker concept among cardiologists at the time. Through a professional organization that brought together doctors and engineers, he met William Chardack, a surgeon at the local Veterans Administration hospital. Chardack encouraged development and in April 1958 the first model cardiac pacemaker was implanted in a dog.[49] Greatbatch worked full time on the device, using his own personal funds to finance the development. In the next two years, working alone in his wood-heated barn, he made fifty pacemakers, ten of which were implanted in human beings.

In 1961, Chardack and Greatbatch collaborated with another electrical engineer, Earl Bakken, who was president of Medtronic, a small Minneapolis company. Medtronic had been formed in 1949 as an outgrowth of the electronic hospital equipment repair business that Bakken began as a graduate student. The selling and servicing of hospital equipment led to requests from physicians to modify equipment or to design and produce products needed for special tests. Among those physician customers was C. Walton Lillehie, a pioneer open-heart surgeon at the University of Minnesota. Lillehie turned to Medtronic to develop a reliable power source for heart stimulation. Bakken developed the first wearable, battery operated external pacemaker in 1958. These external pacemakers, however, were cumbersome, the lead wires to the heart snagged and dislodged, and there was risk of infection where the wires passed through the skin. By late 1960, the team of Bakken and Greatbatch was formed. Medtronic secured exclusive rights to produce and market the Chardack-Greatbatch implantable pacemaker device.

The first clinically successful, self-contained, battery powered pacemaker was implanted in a human being in 1960. Within a decade of their introduction, pacemakers became a useful tool for cardiac patients. But problems with many of the early devices arose, and considerable incremental innovation and development followed. Battery technology improved, in part as a result of NASA supported technology on hermetically sealed, nickel cadmium batteries that could function for years in orbiting spacecraft. The inventor of the first rechargeable cardiac pacemaker formed Pacesetter Systems to manufacture and market the rechargeable battery developed in 1968. Greatbatch worked on the development of lithium batteries, which had considerably greater longevity than earlier ones. Cardiac Pacemakers (CPI) introduced them in 1971. Intermedics entered the market in 1973 with a second lithium battery. Additional problems arose with the lead wire technology, including fracturing and dislodgement. New materials, processes, and designs have been introduced. Medtronic has been the industry leader in electrode tip and lead wire design.[50]

Since its inception, the pacemaker industry has been both highly competitive and highly innovative. The industry is fairly stable; while a number of companies entered early, five companies have dominated the marketplace. Medtronic, the pioneer in pacemakers, has remained the industry leader, holding 42 percent of market share in 1988. Pacesetter Systems was founded in 1970 in a joint effort with the Applied Physics Laboratory of the Johns Hopkins University. In 1985 the company was acquired by Siemens-Elema AB, then a world leader in pacemakers, though it had only a small share of the U.S. market. The buyout gave Siemens-Pacesetter the second position in the current U.S. market.

Another early entrant was CPI, founded in 1971 by a management group formerly associated with Medtronic. The firm was an innovator in lithium iodide battery powered pacemakers, and was acquired by Eli Lilly in 1978. Its market share is about 5 percent. Albert Beutel, a young pacemaker salesman, founded Intermedics in 1974. It started operations as the nation's second largest producer of lithium iodine battery powered pacers and holds a 14 percent market share.[51] Cordis Corporation, which pioneered the programmable pacemakers, recently sold its floundering pacemaker division to Telectronics, a U.S. subsidiary of Australia's Nucleus Limited and one of the world's largest producers of implantable pacemakers. Telectronics took over the manufacturing facility of General Electric in 1976, when that firm withdrew from pacemaker production. Telectronics/Cordis holds a 13 percent market share.

Over the course of the last twelve years, the industry was highly innovative. The earliest devices were single-chamber products with pulse generators permanently preset at the time of implantation. Technological advances included the development of multiprogrammable units that allow the physician to modify the parameters, such as the rate of beats and the level of electrical stimulation, without surgery. Another important innovation was the dual-chamber unit. Dual-chamber devices benefit patients who have a loss of synchrony between the two chambers of the heart. Dual-chamber units represented only 5 percent of implants in 1981 and 23 percent of implants by 1984.[52]

The most recent innovation was the introduction of the rate-responsive pacemaker. Medtronic's Activitrax is the first single-chamber pacemaker that detects body movement and automatically adjusts paced heart rates based on activity. This is accomplished by means of an activity sensing crystal bonded to the inside of the pacemaker's titanium shell. When the crystal is stressed by pressure produced from body activity, it creates a tiny electrical current that signals the pacemaker to change rates. Medtronic received FDA approval in June 1986. Within the first year on the market, rate-responsive pacemakers captured 22 percent of the American market and account for Medtronic's continuing success.[53] (See figure 15.)

There has been additional innovation in lead wire technology. Lead wires link the power source to the heart muscle. Medtronic has been the leader in electrode tip design. Advances in software, sensors to detect and respond to physiologic demands, and microelectronics and batteries to reduce the size and weight of pacemakers continue to advance the usefulness of this medical device for more and more patients.

By the time pacemakers were sophisticated enough to enter the medical marketplace, the Medicare program was well underway. Because the medical conditions that respond to pacemaking generally afflict older people, innovators in this field had a federally subsidized market for their products.

The pacemaker market grew steadily with sales increasing from 60,000 units in 1974, to 80,000 in 1976, and to 114,000 in 1984. Throughout the 1980s, about 85 percent of all pacemaker surgeries were eligible for Medicare reimbursement. In 1984, Medicare paid $775 million to hospitals for pacemaker surgeries, including $400 million for hospital purchases of the

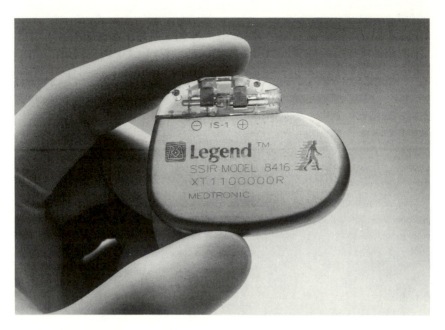

Figure 15. The Medtronic Legend™ pacemaker. Photo courtesy of Medtronic, Inc.

pacemaker devices themselves. Given the role of Medicare, the pacemaker industry is inextricably linked to the government policy that essentially supports the marketplace.[54]

While innovative and competitive, this industry is hardly a model of corporate responsibility. The structure of the federally subsidized market fostered some of the high-pressure sales tactics that led to significant fraud and abuse. Under the Medicare cost-plus system, there was little incentive for hospitals to seek discounts and no incentive to get warranty credits when a pacemaker under warranty failed. Companies began rapacious competition on nonprice attributes. A 1981 report stated that "the absence of price competition as a significant factor in the domestic market has, of course, spawned the kind of competitive environment that exists today. The cardiologist or surgeon who makes the product decision is insensitive to price since the pacemaker . . . is reimbursable by various health insurance programs."[55]

There were roughly 500–550 salespeople for only 1,500 physicians that implanted pacemakers. An article in *Medical World News* in September 1982 reported that companies were offering physicians free vacations, stock options at reduced prices, cash kickbacks, and consulting jobs with liberal compensation to persuade them to use the products.[56] Companies instituted sales incentive programs to encourage unnecessary implantations, as well as unnecessary explantations and reinsertions of new products.

The Senate Special Committee on Aging held hearings in 1982 to investigate the industry. One disgruntled former salesman summed up the situation: "In all my twenty years experience in the medical sales field, I have never seen a business so dirty, so immensely profitable, and so absent normal competitive price controls as this one."[57] The General Accounting Office undertook a study of the situation as a result of the 1982 hearings, and Congress held follow-up hearings in 1985.[58] By then, however, Medicare cost controls had been instituted, and the hospital purchasing environment had changed. In an effort to control costs generally, the HCFA instituted oversight and price-setting controls. The GAO found that PPS had given hospitals financial incentives to be more cost-conscious purchasers. Clearly the pacemaker producers would feel the pinch as price became an important attribute in pacemaker purchasing decisions.

Other companies encountered criminal problems. On 12 October 1983, Pacesetter Systems was indicted on four counts of offering to pay and paying kickbacks and one count of conspiracy. Company officials pleaded guilty to charges, and its former president pleaded nolo contendere. On 6 July 1984, Telectronics pleaded guilty to four counts of having paid kickbacks to a cardiologist. The FBI also uncovered more sophisticated kickback schemes.[59] Cordis, unsullied in the 1982 congressional investigations, pleaded guilty in 1988 to multiple federal charges that it sold pacemakers it knew were faulty.[60] A federal judge rejected the plea agreement with the government in which Cordis would have paid a $123,000 fine, saying that "the . . . fine simply is not commensurate with the crime." In April 1989 Cordis pleaded guilty to twenty-five criminal violations, including thirteen felony counts. Cordis agreed to pay the maximum fine of $623,000, plus $141,000 to reimburse the government for its in-

vestigative costs, and to pay $5 million for the civil fraud of sell-
ing defective pacemakers to the VA and the DHHS. Four former
executives also faced trial in 1989 on forty-three counts.[61] Medtronic settled for $3 million with the government to reimburse
Medicare for replacement of defective pacemaker leads.[62]

It is clear that the Medicare program, per se, did not cause the
abusive practices in some pacemaker companies. However, the
availability of reimbursement dollars promoted an atmosphere
of non-price competition that encouraged less scrupulous companies. More recent efforts to establish oversight and financial
incentive for hospitals have begun to change the environment.
Medicare's lack of controls must take some responsibility for the
abuses.

CONCLUSION

The three technologies presented here represent important
medical products. Countless lives have been saved by kidney
dialysis. More accurate diagnosis through the CT scanner benefits all patients. The quality of life for heart patients is improved
by implanted pacemakers. These cases are representative of
many medical devices appearing on the market in the 1960s and
1970s. Public policy promoted the distribution of medical devices. In an era when costs were relatively unimportant and few
restraints on acquisition existed, devices had potentially large
markets. From an industry perspective, this was a golden age for
device innovation. Until the 1970s, the prescriptions for our
patient—the medical device industry—fueled growth and development at the discovery and the distribution stage.

However, we have seen that unrestrained industry growth is
not necessarily socially desirable. Abuses occurred in both Medicare and Medicaid programs. This golden age for device producers could not and did not last. Early efforts to contain costs
and slow diffusion appeared by the mid-1970s. Concern about
safety led to expansion of FDA regulation. New prescriptions
were needed to keep the patient in its place. We now turn to
these new efforts to control and inhibit device technology.

5

GOVERNMENT INHIBITS
MEDICAL DEVICE DISCOVERY:
REGULATION

	Discovery	Distribution
Promote	1. National Institutes of Health (NIH) Space & Defense Spinoffs	2. Hill-Burton Hospital Construction Funds Medicare/Medicaid
Inhibit	3. Regulation (FDA) Product Liability	4. Certificate of Need Cost-Containment Technology Assessment

Figure 16. The policy matrix.

The policies discussed in chapters 3 and 4 changed American medicine. Neither was designed specifically to promote the medical device industry; federal R&D was primarily directed at biomedical research, and federal and state payment programs were designed to increase access to health care. Nevertheless, the medical device industry benefited. Increasingly sophisticated devices became available to large numbers of people. Devices began to lose their association with quack products and were frequently linked to therapeutic breakthroughs.

However, many of these sophisticated new technologies, such as pacemakers, kidney dialysis equipment, and diagnostic instruments, presented risks along with their potential benefits. Adverse effects associated with cardiac pacemakers, intrauterine devices (IUDs), and implanted interocular lenses, in particular, raised public concern.

The ground was fertile for federal regulation of these products. The late 1960s and the 1970s were a time of growing consumer activism and power. Product safety became a desirable value that the federal government was expected to protect. The government was expanding safety regulation in many new areas, including consumer products, the workplace, and the environment. In many instances, Congress created new regulatory agencies to address safety issues, including the Environmental Protection Agency (1969), the Occupational Safety and Health Administration (1972), and the Consumer Product Safety Commission (1972). In the case of medical devices, the FDA was already in place with expertise and some preexisting jurisdiction over the industry.

This chapter describes the political process leading to the expanded regulation of medical devices, the first major legislation directed exclusively at the device industry. (See figure 16.) Issues related to the structure and implementation of the Medical Device Amendments of 1976 are discussed, illustrated by cases such as IUDs, lithotripsy equipment, pacemaker components, and tampons.

Once again, a brief caveat before proceeding. By the 1970s, the effects of policy proliferation became apparent. For example, the impact of some regulation was blunted by the Medicare policies that encouraged purchases regardless of cost. Thus costs associated with regulation could be passed along without concern. For other products, the interaction with regulation and product liability increased environmental threats. Issues relating to product liability are discussed fully in chapter 6.

MEDICAL DEVICE REGULATION COMES OF AGE

The Limitations of FDA Authority

As we saw in chapter 2, the FDA had very limited powers over medical devices under the 1938 Food, Drug, and Cosmetic Act. Its primary authority was seizure of individual devices found to be adulterated or misbranded. Most of the FDA's early enforcement activity was directed toward controlling obvious quack devices. However, even this limited regulatory activity declined during World War II. Because of the scarcity of metals and other critical materials, production of nonessential devices was restricted, and consequently the pace of seizures and prosecutions dropped to less than six per year.[1]

After World War II, there was an increase in device quackery because of the cheap availability of war surplus electrical and electronic equipment.[2] A variety of products that used dangerous gases (such as ozone and chlorine), radio waves, heat, and massage were marketed for the treatment of almost every disease known. Among the most dangerous were quack devices that used radium, uranium ore, and other radioactive substances and that purported to cure common problems such as sinus infections and arthritis.

The pace of FDA seizures picked up in response. In a report in 1963, the Bureau of Enforcement of the FDA's Device Division stated that from 1961 to 1963, the FDA seized 111 different types of misbranded or worthless devices, involving 15,070 individual units. Fifty-four diagnostic and treatment devices were taken in 358 seizure actions from June 1962 to June 1963.[3] Some states tried to tackle the problem with their own legislation. For example, California had passed a state Pure Foods and Drug Act in 1907, one year after the first federal act. The law prohibited any claim for a food, drug, or device that was false or misleading in any particular. California brought over sixty court actions from 1948 to 1957. The focus of this early activity was on fraudulent devices; concern about the safety of clearly therapeutic products came later.[4]

Congressional legislative activity focused on drug risks in the late 1960s. Congress increased FDA power to regulate drugs in 1962 in response to controversial evidence linking birth defects and the drug thalidomide.[5] The 1962 amendments to the Food, Drug, and Cosmetic Act greatly strengthened federal power over drugs by requiring proof that the product was both safe and efficacious before it received FDA marketing approval. Because of the previous distinction between drugs and devices made in the 1938 law, these expanded powers did not apply to new medical devices.[6]

By the late 1960s, problems associated with legitimate, thera-
peutically desirable medical devices that were flooding the marketplace began to surface. In 1970, Dr. Theodore Cooper, then
director of the NIH Heart and Lung Institute, completed a survey of the previous ten years that revealed 10,000 injuries from
medical devices, including 731 deaths. Defective heart valves
caused 512 of the deaths.[7] In particular, problems had arisen
involving defective pacemakers[8] and intrauterine devices.[9] Congress, the FDA, and the public became concerned.

Creative Regulation by the FDA

The increase in legitimate medical devices complicated the
FDA's regulatory efforts. The sophisticated new technologies,
such as pacemakers, kidney dialysis units, cardiac, renal, and
other catheters, surgical implants, and diagnostic instruments,
challenged the FDA's expertise. The agency's regulatory power
was limited to seizure of products already on the market. In
order to bring a seizure action under the law, the FDA had to
consult experts, sponsor research, and gather data to meet its
statutory burden of proof in court. The real problem was that
seizures were simply not a reasonable response to devices that
had benefits as well as risks. The goal was not to remove these
products from the market as much as to ensure that these innovations were safe.

In the absence of additional authority, the FDA began to
implement the law more aggressively. One tactic was to construe
the statutory definition of *drug* broadly enough to include products that were clearly medical devices and thus would allow the
agency to regulate devices much as it regulated drugs.

Device companies challenged this effort to impose drug regulation on devices. Two important court decisions in the late
1960s upheld the FDA's broad reading of the term *drug*. In *AMP
v. Gardner*, the court reviewed the FDA's classification as a "new
drug" a nylon binding device used to tie off severed blood vessels
during surgery.[10] The court broadly construed the purpose of
the 1938 act and the 1962 amendments, holding that the goal
was to keep inadequately tested and potentially harmful "medical products" out of interstate commerce. Emphasizing the pro-

tective purposes of the law enabled the government to regulate as a drug any product not generally recognized as safe.

The next year, the Supreme Court followed similar reasoning in *United States v. An Article of Drug . . . Bacto-Unidisk.* [11] In 1960, after the product had been in use for four years, the secretary of HEW classified an antibiotic disk as a drug. The product, which never came into contact with the human body and was therefore not metabolized, was used as a screening test in a laboratory to determine the proper antibiotic to administer. Its classification as a drug came after the agency received numerous complaints from the medical profession, hospitals, and laboratory technicians that the statements of potency for the disks were unreliable. The FDA found it "vital for the protection of public health" to adopt the regulations.[12]

The Court, acknowledging that the FDA was an expert agency charged with the enforcement of remedial regulation, deferred to the secretary's medical judgment. It concluded that the term *drug* was a legal term of art for purposes of the law, which was a broader interpretation than the strict medical definition. The Court determined that the parallel definitions of drugs and devices, discussed previously, was "semantic." Concluding that there was no "practical significance to the distinction" until subsequent amendments to the 1938 Act, the Court gave the term "a liberal construction consistent with the act's overriding purpose to protect public health."[13]

IUDs

The FDA's response to problems associated with implanted intrauterine devices illustrates its efforts to regulate creatively to protect the public. IUDs to prevent pregnancy had been available since the turn of the century. Although they had been generally dismissed as dangerous by respectable practitioners, the technology began to be reevaluated in the late 1950s. The renewed interest in contraceptives, the availability of inert plastics that caused fewer tissue reactions, and the growing controversies about the safety of the new contraceptive pills all encouraged research on IUDs.

IUD devices began to enter the market in the mid-1960s.

From 1969 to the early 1970s, IUD use skyrocketed. By the end of 1970, three million women in the United States had been fitted with a variety of IUD devices. Marketing was aggressive, and the competition among firms was keen. The top sellers included Ortho Pharmaceutical's Lippes Loop, the Saf-T-Coil produced by Schmidt Labs, and the now infamous Dalkon Shield introduced by A. H. Robins in January 1971.[14] G. D. Searle entered the market in the same year with the Cu-7, a device shaped like the number 7 with a small thread of copper wound around the vertical arm, which the company claimed increased the product's efficacy. The data regarding unit sales testify to the early success of these products (see table 6).

Despite burgeoning sales, product safety remained a concern. As early as 1968, an FDA advisory committee on obstetrics and gynecology cited significant injuries and some deaths associated with IUDs.[15] The devices generated numerous complaints, and there were reports of infections, sterility, and, on some occasions, death.

Under the device provisions of the 1938 law, the FDA had only the limited power to seize individual products, an impractical remedy in this situation. An internal FDA memorandum recommended that the *AMP v. Gardner* precedent be used to designate all products intended for prolonged internal use to be considered "drugs" for purposes of premarket approval.[16] If this recommendation had been adopted, all implanted devices, including pacemakers and IUDs, would have been officially considered drugs under the law.

The agency did not go so far. In 1971 it considered a proposed rule on the classification of IUDs. At that time, G. D. Searle began to market the Cu-7 IUD. Because this device contained a noninert substance, the FDA's final rule in 1973 distinguished between device-type IUDs and drug IUDs. The agency treated as a regulated drug any IUD that contained heavy metals or any substance that might be biologically active in the body. An IUD was a device, hence exempt from premarket approval requirements, if it was fabricated entirely from inactive materials or if substances "added to improve the physical characteristics [did] not contribute to contraception through chemical action on or within the body."[17] Thus, Searle's Cu-7 was subjected

Table 6. Numbers of IUDs Sold

Year	Dalkon Shield	Saf-T-Coil	Lippes Loop
1971	1,081,000	180,060	409,176
1972	883,500	178,995	411,952
1973	604,400	230,561	492,912

Source: Morton Mintz, *At Any Cost: Corporate Greed, Women, and the Dalkon Shield* (New York: Pantheon, 1985), 281.

to premarket approval, as was Progestasert, an IUD with a timed-release contraceptive hormone that entered the market in 1976.

FDA officials later admitted the frustration of using the drug provisions as a substitute for adequate device regulation. Despite efforts to increase the staff for the Medical Devices Program, the agency had limited resources for the regulation of devices as drugs.[18] Other important jurisdictional issues arose as well. In 1972, Peter Barton Hutt, general counsel for the FDA, said that "The administrative burden of handling all devices under the new drug provisions of the act would be overwhelming. . . . If we were to reclassify all devices as new drugs, difficult legal issues would be raised about our authority to allow them to remain on the market pending approval of an NDA [new drug approval]. Wholesale removal of marketed products would, of course, not be medically warranted."[19] Without clear legislative authority, the FDA was unwilling to regulate devices through use of the provisions intended to apply only to drugs.

As might be expected, problems related to devices continued to arise. When reports of severe adverse reactions were specifically associated with the Dalkon Shield, an advisor to the FDA recommended that it be removed from the market. The big question was how to do so under the law. The only power the FDA had was to get a court injunction to halt interstate shipments of adulterated and misbranded products and to proceed to seize them one at a time. Of course, for implanted products, safety would clearly be better served by preventing these products from entering the market in the first place. A. H. Robins finally admitted the inevitability of some government action, and, in the wake of significant adverse publicity, the company voluntarily suspended sales, pending a hearing of FDA advisory bodies. The product never returned to the market.[20] The FDA ultimately got the outcome it desired, but its formal regulatory impotence did not go unnoticed by Congress or the public.

Congress Takes Action

The limited powers of the FDA had been graphically demonstrated during the Dalkon Shield controversy. Congress not only was aware of the publicity concerning harmful devices but also had held hearings on several products during this period.[21] Bills to expand the FDA's authority over devices had been introduced every year from 1969 to 1975. The likelihood of congressional action was increased by the fact that consumer activism was at its peak. The controversies surrounding IUDs mobilized the nascent women's movement, and defective cardiac pacemakers caused concern among the elderly. Ralph Nader's Health Research Group vigorously lobbied government to protect consumers in the areas of medicine and health products.

On the other side, the medical device industry was not well organized. Until this time, government had been either neutral or a benefactor, not a threat to the industry's well-being. In fact, there was no trade association until the mid-1970s. Unlike the drug industry, which was represented by the old and powerful Pharmaceutical Manufacturers Association (PMA), the device producers were a disparate group with no clearly identifiable or shared issues. Many were small innovators with little or no experience with the political process.

The prospect of regulation spurred organizing efforts. The Health Industry Manufacturers Association (HIMA) formed in 1976, but it was too late to stop Congress from regulating the industry. Indeed, the organization was established in direct response to the new regulatory threat. Some larger device companies had their own Washington offices that handled government relations; for smaller companies, HIMA was the only representation. HIMA has since become larger and more active, but in the 1970s members of the industry were reactive, not proactive. Regulation was only a matter of time.

The Medical Device Amendments of 1976

The Medical Device Amendments of 1976 sought to provide "reasonable assurance of safety and effectiveness" for all devices.[22] The FDA was to determine whether such assurance existed by "weighing any probable benefit to health from the use of the device against any probable risk of injury or illness from such use." The law conferred powers upon the FDA to regulate medical devices during all phases of development, testing, production, distribution, and use.

In order to accomplish these goals, Congress devised a complicated regulatory scheme. This complexity arose from both the diversity of the products to be regulated and the lack of trust between Congress and the FDA at that time. The diversity of devices dictated a regulatory system that would provide levels of government scrutiny appropriate to the nature of each device. The lack of trust meant that Congress did not give the agency discretion to implement the law; instead, detailed provisions were intended to force the agency to regulate with vigor.[23]

In the law, Congress used two different methods to group medical devices: first, devices were divided into three classes on the basis of risk, with increasing rigor from Class I to Class III; and second, they were divided into seven categories (preamendment, postamendment, substantially equivalent, implant, custom, investigational, and transitional). It is not surprising that a complicated system emerged from these numerous divisions.

In brief, Class I, general controls, is the least regulated class, and it requires producers to comply with regulations on registration, premarketing notice, record keeping, labeling, reporting of adverse experiences, and good manufacturing processes. These controls apply to all three classes of devices. Manufacturers of Class I devices must register their establishments and list their devices with the FDA and notify it at least ninety days before they intend to market a device. Tongue depressors are an example of a Class I device. Class II devices are those for which general controls are considered insufficient to ensure safety and effectiveness and for which information exists to establish performance standards. Well over half of the devices on the market are in Class II.

Class III consists of those devices for which general controls alone are insufficient to ensure safety and efficacy and for which information does not exist to establish a performance standard *and* the device supports life, prevents health impairment, or presents a potentially unreasonable risk of illness or injury. Only those devices placed in Class III receive premarket reviews similar to those conducted on drugs. The manufacturer must submit a premarket approval application (PMA) that provides sufficient data to assure the FDA that the device is safe and efficacious. Only a small fraction (about 8 percent) of all devices are placed in Class III, including heart valves and other implanted products.

The categories set forth in the law established guidelines for classification. For example, implanted devices are assumed to require a Class III placement, and custom and investigational devices can be exempt from premarket testing and performance standards. Examples of implants include cardiac pacemakers and artificial hips; custom devices include dentures and orthopedic shoes; and at present investigational devices include the artificial heart and positron emission tomography (PET) imaging machines. Transitional devices are those regulated as drugs (such as copper-based IUDs) before the passage of the law, and they are automatically assigned to Class III. Devices on the market at the time the law was passed are referred to as *preamendment* or *preenactment devices*. These products are assumed to be in Class I unless their safety and efficacy cannot be ensured without more regulation. Manufacturers can petition for reclassification under certain circumstances.

One provision has assumed a greater significance in practice than was perceived when the law was drafted. New devices that are shown to be "substantially equivalent" to a device on the market before the law was passed are assigned to the same class as their earlier counterparts, and manufacturers have to provide information on testing and approval only if the earlier products required it. To receive the designation of substantial equivalence, section 510k requires producers to notify the FDA at least ninety days before marketing. This premarket notification must contain enough information for the FDA to determine whether the device is substantially equivalent to a device already being marketed.[24] A product need not be identical, but it cannot differ markedly in design or materials. If a device meets the equivalence requirement, it can go directly to market without further scrutiny. The benefits to manufacturers of "a 510k" are enormous, as their products can enter the market quickly and without great effort.

This complex regulatory framework invites maneuvering on the part of producers. Unlike the drug law that treats all new chemical entities (NCEs) alike, the medical device amendments present a large number of options and opportunities to manipulate the system. The FDA's management of the device law has been very controversial. Frequent hearings and investigations by Congress have tended to conclude that the FDA has not measured up.[25] On the other hand, some in industry have accused the FDA of overregulation, inefficiency, and harassment. For its part, the FDA claims that limited resources and expanding demands hamper enforcement.

IMPLEMENTATION OF THE FDA'S NEW POWERS

FDA authority over the device industry falls into two general categories—barriers to market entry (premarket controls) and the power to oversee production of a marketed product or to remove it from the marketplace (postmarket controls). Issues of implementation have arisen in both categories.

Premarket Controls:
Problems of Classification and Categorization

The classification of the device determines the level of scrutiny it receives. The ability of the law to reduce risks depends upon a rational classification process. If barriers are too high, desirable innovations will be discouraged. If they are too low, the public will not receive the protection the law intended. Given the number of vastly different devices subject to regulation and the limited resources and energy of the agency, there are many problems regarding classifications.

Because the degree of regulation varies significantly depending on the classification of a device, it is not surprising that there have been disputes over how the FDA evaluates industry petitions to reclassify a device. An important set of judicial opinions clarified the FDA's authority to deny reclassification petitions.

Two appellate court decisions in the D.C. Circuit Court of Appeals affirmed the FDA's discretion to deny reclassification petitions if it finds insufficient scientific evidence to do so. In *Contact Lens Manufacturers Association v. FDA*,[26] the trade association challenged the FDA's refusal to reclassify rigid gas-permeable lenses (RGP) from Class III to Class I. Hard contact lenses (polymethylmethacrylate, or PMMA) have been marketed in the United States since the early 1950s. Soft lenses (hydroxyethylmethacrylate, or HEMA) lenses are a more recent development. In September 1975, citing their "novelty," the FDA announced that all HEMA lenses would be regarded as "new drugs" and regulated as such. Upon passage of the Medical Device Amendments, all devices regulated as drugs were automatically in Class III under a "transitional" device provision.[27] In 1981, the FDA considered reclassification of RGP lenses, a type of soft lens, into Class I, which would greatly have reduced regulatory oversight. However, after receiving extensive comments, the FDA withdrew its proposed reclassification,[28] and the industry association petitioned the court for review of the FDA's power. The court upheld the FDA's authority to withdraw its proposal. In *General Medical v. FDA*[29] the court upheld the FDA's decision to deny a petition for reclassification of the Drionic device, a product used to prevent excessive perspiration.

Additional problems have arisen regarding devices on the market before the passage of the law. Many of these devices are considered Class III, but they have been largely ignored. The first premarket approval application (PMA) for a preenactment device was not required until June 1984, a full eight years after the law had been passed. The FDA stated that the implanted cerebellar stimulator was chosen because of contradictory information about its effectiveness for some indications.[30] In 1983, the FDA published a notice of intent to require premarketing approval of twelve other preenactment devices.[31] After years of controversy, the FDA finally required PMAs for preenactment heart valves in June 1987.

The FDA has also been criticized for its failure to implement the Class II requirements. Class II devices are supposed to meet performance standards to ensure safety and efficacy. The statutory provisions for the selection of a standard-setting body and the drafting of standards are exceedingly detailed.[32] The process itself would be costly and slow, arguably locking in the state of the art at the time a standard was set. More than 50 percent of the 1,700 classified types of devices are in Class II, but not one performance standard had been issued by 1988.[33] Given that performance standards are the only distinction between Class II and Class I, this situation makes a mockery of the classification system.

Premarket Notification: Pacemaker Leads

Problems related to pacemaker leads illustrate the controversy surrounding 510k, the provision for premarket notification as a substitute for FDA review. Pacemaker leads connect a pacemaker's power source to the heart muscle itself. Innovators have had many problems with lead design—leads tend to become dislodged and render the pacing device ineffective. Many new designs emerged as the pacemaker industry developed, and there were a significant number of lead failures.

Congress held hearings in 1984 on the Medtronic polyurethane pacemaker leads. The congressional inquiry was prompted by reports that certain Medtronic pacemaker leads failed at abnormally high rates—about 10 percent or greater by the third year after implantation. There was much concern about the history and status of Medtronic's premarket notification (510k) submissions for polyurethane leads; major manufacturing and design changes that could affect the safety and effectiveness of their leads occurred without any FDA premarket scrutiny. Lead innovations had been designated "substantially equivalent" because leads performed the same function as the earlier products, but these were clearly very different in design, materials, and structure from their predecessors.

The FDA subsequently modified its procedures for reviewing premarket notification applications because of its experiences with Medtronic. By the mid-1980s, FDA required more evidence of comparable safety and effectiveness to support substantial equivalence decisions: results of all types of testing, more elaborate statistical analyses of test data, and, for cardiovascular devices that are life-supporting, life-sustaining, or implanted, summaries of equivalence similar to summaries of safety and effectiveness required for premarket approval.[34] The underlying premise for 510k procedures was that a product was substantially similar to one on the market, and presumably its safety and efficacy had already been determined. It is fundamentally inconsistent to have innovative design and manufacturing changes enter the market in this fashion. After over a decade, the FDA finally began to rectify the problem.

The Burdens of Class III: The Case of Extracorporeal Shock-wave Lithotripsy

Only a very small percentage of devices are placed in Class III and therefore are subject to the full premarket review similar to drug evaluations. This process can be extremely time-consuming and expensive for the producer. Of course, the purpose is to produce sufficient safety and efficacy data to ensure that the product meets the statutory standards before entering the market. The introduction of extracorporeal shock-wave lithotripsy (ESWL) in 1984 illustrates dynamic innovation in the private sector and its interrelationship with regulation.

Kidney stones in the urinary tract (urolithiasis) develop when minerals, primarily calcium and oxalate, form crystals rather than being diluted and passed out of the body. More than 300,000 patients a year (70 percent of them young to middle-aged males) develop kidney stones. For many, treatment with fluids and painkillers is sufficient; for 20 to 40 percent, the stones cause infections, impaired kidney function, or severe pain and warrant more aggressive intervention. Until the last decade, surgery to remove the stones was the only form of medical help for severe kidney stone problems.[35]

The first major advance was in the early 1980s. Percutaneous endoscopic techniques permitted a physician to make a small incision and attempt stone extraction or disintegration using a special scope. The second major advance was ESWL. Its most exciting feature was that it offered a noninvasive way to treat kidney stones. The first ESWL devices required the patient to be placed in a water bath. After X-ray monitors positioned the patient, a high-voltage underwater spark generated intense sound waves. The resultant waves disintegrated the stone into fine bits of sand that could easily pass out of the body. (The term *lithotripsy* comes from classical Greek and means "stone crushing."[36]) Subsequent technological modifications eliminated the need for the water bath, and mobile units were developed. Devices that use optical fibers as conduits for laser light pulses that fragment the stones are currently in experimental stages of development.[37]

While ESWL is an exciting innovation, several factors might have led to skepticism about its likely commercial success. The equipment was very expensive (early models cost at least $1.5 million), there was a viable surgical alternative, and the patient base was small and likely to remain so. And because the device was in Class III, it was subject to the highest level of premarket scrutiny.[38]

The product took thirteen months to receive FDA approval, slightly longer than the average of one year. Despite this delay to market, it diffused rapidly once available. There were over two hundred lithotripters in operation within two years of introduction (see figure 17). The market now includes 220 devices and is basically saturated. Of ten firms in the market, only four have received FDA approval; the others have devices in investigational stages (see table 7). The market leader is Dornier Medical Systems, the first to receive a PMA; the others include Medstone International, Diasonics, Technomed International, and Northgate Research.[39]

The next generation of machines is already in development. In a relatively short time, there have been major improvements in the original device; other designs, such as those that use laser technology, are on the horizon. There have been a number of creative marketing solutions to the problems of high cost and low patient volume. Entrepreneurs have put together joint ventures with physicians and hospitals that ensure a broad patient base, lower the unit cost of treatment, and amortize the cost of the device. Some free-standing centers have developed relationships with providers of other forms of kidney stone treatment so

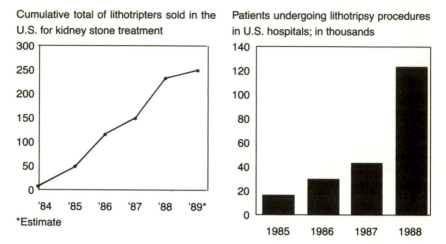

Cumulative total of lithotripters sold in the U.S. for kidney stone treatment

Patients undergoing lithotripsy procedures in U.S. hospitals; in thousands

*Estimate

Figure 17. Treating kidney stones with shock waves. Adapted from Ron Winslow, "Costly Shock-wave Machines Fare Poorly on Gallstones," *Wall Street Journal,* 9 February 1991, B1.

that comprehensive services and alternative treatments to lithotripsy are all available in one location.[40]

What lessons can we learn from this case about the nature of innovation in the device industry? How can we explain the success of this expensive, highly regulated technology? One possible explanation is that promising and truly useful technologies usually succeed despite the barriers placed in their paths. However, it may be that the dynamism and creativity are based on the expectation of enormous market expansion through the application of this technology to patients with gallstones, a much more prevalent clinical condition than kidney stones. There are 20 million gallstone patients in the United States, with 487,000 gall bladder removals in hospitals every year. Medicare plays an important role because gallstone disease affects many elderly people. The treatment of gallbladder disease is a $5 billion market. If lithotripsy could be applied to some of these patients, hospitals could avoid many of the surgical costs and the firms could compete for this greatly expanded market.[41] (See figure 18.)

Whether that expansion will occur is now in doubt, and here is where the policy process reenters. In October 1989, an FDA advisory panel recommended that the agency disapprove the PMAs filed by Dornier Medical Systems and Medstone International for gallstone (biliary) lithotripters. The panel members expressed concern about the safety data in the PMAs. Questions were also raised about the effectiveness of lithotripsy for destroying all gallstones. Preliminary evaluations revealed that only a small percentage of patients with gallstones may benefit from EWSL.[42]

The delay (or possible denial) in marketing approval may allow competitors to catch up with the two leaders, although the ultimate clinical usefulness of biliary lithotripsy remains uncertain. Manufacturers have been slow to gather sufficient data because the lack of any third-party reimbursement for this new procedure has limited the number of patients who have received it. In addition, because the drugs used in conjunction with the treatment work slowly, studies are often time-consuming. In the meantime, alternative treatments are developing, including a laser that views and snips off the gallbladder and pulls it out through a small incision. Other experiments include a rotary device that whips gallstones until they liquefy and then draws out the resulting "soup."[43]

The failure of biliary lithotripters to receive FDA approval may only be a temporary and minor delay. It may also indicate that the technology is inappropriate for the proposed use, and the FDA is sagely valuing safety concerns over the desires of the innovative firms to rush to market. Or we may be seeing a regulatory failure in which the FDA is inappropriately obstructing a valuable innovation from the marketplace. The FDA's decision delays reimbursement from third-party payers, including Medicare, which will rarely pay for unapproved technologies, further burdening the innovators. The FDA approval does not necessarily guarantee Medicare's coverage of the procedure. The Health Care Financing Administration (HCFA), Medicare's payment authority, makes its own assessments of new technologies for coverage and payment decisions, often independently of FDA findings.[44]

The lithotripsy industry remains dynamic, highly innovative, and very competitive. However, the market for kidney stone treatment is saturated and not expanding. No improved

Table 7. Lithotripter Manufacturers

Company	Machine	Price	Shock-wave Generator	Shock-wave Coupling	Imaging Method	FDA Status	Mobile
Diasonics	Therasonic	$1M	Ultrasonic	Membrane	X-ray, ultrasound	PMA submitted— renal IDE biliary	Yes
Direx	Tripter XI	$400,000	Spark gap	Membrane	NA (can upgrade to ultrasound)	IDE renal pending IDE biliary	Yes
Dornier Medical Systems	MFL 5000 HM4 MPL9000	NA $1.5M NA	Spark gap Spark gap Spark gap	Membrane Membrane Membrane	X-ray X-ray X-ray, ultrasound	IDE renal PMA renal IDE biliary, renal	Yes Yes Yes
EDAP International	LITHEDAP LT.01	$990,000	Piezoelectric	Membrane	Ultrasound	IDE renal IDE biliary	Yes
Medstone International	STS	$1.4M	Spark gap	Membrane	X-ray, ultrasound	PMA renal IDE biliary	Yes

Company	Model	Price	Generator	Coupling	Imaging	Status	In U.S.?
Northgate Research	SD-3	$650,000	Spark gap	Membrane	Ultrasound	pending PMA renal IDE biliary	
Richard Wolf Medical Instruments	Piezolith 2300	$1M–1.5M	Piezoelectric	Water basin	X-ray, ultrasound	PMA filed renal IDE biliary	Yes
Siemens Medical Systems	Lithostar	$1.2M	Electromagnetic	Membrane	X-ray	PMA renal	Yes
	Lithostar Plus	$1.5M	Electromagnetic	Membrane	X-ray, ultrasound	IDE biliary	Yes
Karl Storz Endoscopy America	Modulith SL10	NA	Electromagnetic	Membrane	X-ray, ultrasound	NA	No
Technomed International	Sonolith 3000	$1.2M	Spark gap	Water basin	Ultrasound	PMA renal pending IDE biliary	Yes

Source: Healthweek, 4 December 1989, 21.

IDE = Investigational Device Exemption allows expanded clinical testing.

PMA = Premarketing approval.

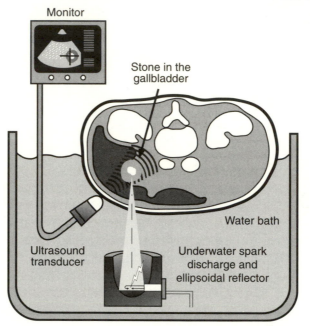

Figure 18. Electrohydraulic shock-wave
lithotripter.
Source: Healthweek, 4 December 1989, 25.

technology to date has left competitors outmoded. Whether the
expansion for use in gallstone treatment will occur depends
upon the public sector—the FDA and Medicare—as well as
private third-party payers. The layering effect becomes important here because if the FDA has not approved a treatment, then
the HCFA will not cover it. And, even if the procedure has been
FDA approved, approval does not ensure private or public sector third-party payment.

Postmarket Controls: Reporting Failures

The postmarket surveillance system has four main components:
(1) voluntary reporting of problems from users, such as doctors
or hospitals to the FDA, manufacturers, and others; (2) mandatory reporting of known problems by manufacturers to the
FDA; (3) monitoring and analysis of problems by the FDA; and

(4) a recall process to correct products or remove them from the market.[45]

Significant controversy has surrounded the reporting requirements. Until 1984, the reporting of adverse effects associated with medical devices was voluntary. The FDA received reports from physicians, hospitals, and manufacturers, and these data were entered into the FDA's Device Experience Network (DEN). Investigations revealed that adverse reactions were seriously underreported.[46]

The FDA promulgated a mandatory medical device reporting rule (MDR) that went into effect in December 1984. The key element in the rule is that manufacturers and importers must report to the FDA when they receive or otherwise become aware of information that reasonably suggests that a product has caused or contributed to serious injury or death, or has malfunctioned and is likely to cause harm if the malfunction recurs. There are tight time frames for reporting. In general, an injury is considered serious if it is life-threatening or results in permanent impairment of a bodily function or permanent damage to body structure. Users such as hospitals and doctors can report voluntarily, but they are not required to do so.[47] Serious problems that came to light through MDR were burns related to the misuse of apnea monitors and early depletion of batteries for portable defibrillators.

From the FDA's perspective, MDR also serves as a barometer of trends of adverse product performance. The FDA has received 18,000 MDR reports since the regulation became effective. Eighteen cardiovascular, anesthesiology, and general hospital devices have accounted for 70 percent of the reports.

There has been a great deal of criticism of MDR from the industry, which has argued that the system forces overreporting because of the breadth of the definitions and the short time frame.[48] On the other hand, some health advocates maintain that the reporting system is hampered by the lack of FDA jurisdiction over hospitals and physicians, neither of which can be ordered to report malfunctions. Recent GAO studies of the FDA device recalls (removal from the market of a product that violates FDA laws) found that only half of all recalls had an MDR report associated with them. The FDA became aware of the majority of device problems in ways other than through the required reports, and it did not have reports available in the majority of cases when decisions about health hazards were made. The GAO concluded that "this suggests that the reports have not served as an effective 'early warning' of device problems serious enough to warrant a recall."[49]

Congress conducted further investigations into reporting failures in late 1989. At a hearing held by the House Subcommittee on Health and the Environment, Congressman Sikorski excoriated manufacturers who failed to report hazards associated with their products. Citing GAO statistics, he noted that 48 percent of high-risk products that had been recalled had never reported problems to the FDA. Grieving parents also explained that their son died because an infant monitoring system failed to notify them that he was not breathing.[50]

The comptroller general testified that the GAO had investigated all major components of the postmarket surveillance system since 1986. It found that the FDA was receiving more information than it previously had, but it also noted that the degree of compliance with MDR could not be established, that the FDA's data-processing system was not adequate to handle the reports it did receive, and that the results of the analyses were often not definitive.[51] Thus the controversy over the FDA's ability to perform its duties under the law continued into the 1990s.

Informal Powers

It is important to remember, however, that a federal agency like the FDA need not always initiate formal action to get results. Although there have been substantial problems with reporting requirements, the FDA has exercised its other postmarketing surveillance powers effectively—and often behind the scenes. The case of toxic shock syndrome illustrates this point. It is particularly striking to compare the FDA's informal power in this case to the Dalkon Shield recall in 1976, before the passage of the device law. When problems arose relating to the Dalkon Shield, the FDA had no clear authority to order a product recall.

When the toxic shock crisis arose in the early 1980s, a very different FDA, with a larger stock of potential tools, took charge.

Tampons were introduced in the 1930s and the Tampax brand dominated the market for decades. In the 1970s, Playtex, Johnson & Johnson, and Kimberly Clark marketed tampon varieties. Procter & Gamble, the large consumer product company, entered the market in late 1979. After a $75 million massive media and direct marketing campaign in late 1979, its Rely brand had acquired a 20 percent share of the billion-dollar industry.[52]

Toxic shock syndrome (TSS) is a rare and mysterious disease characterized by high fever, rash, nervous disorders, and potentially fatal physiologic shock. TSS was not initially associated with tampon use. In January 1980, epidemiologists from Minnesota and Wisconsin reported a total of twelve TSS cases to the federal Centers for Disease Control (CDC). The data revealed surprising patterns—all patients were women using tampons. Through that spring, the CDC received additional reports from many states. Following a retrospective case study in May 1980, tampon manufacturers were made aware of the hazards tentatively associated with their products. There were many unanswered medical questions, but because millions of women used tampons, there was fear of potential widespread injuries. In a study of fifty women who had TSS in September 1980, the CDC revealed that 71 percent of those surveyed had used the Rely brand. Procter & Gamble officials immediately defended the product. Within a week, however, they suspended sales of Rely and signed a comprehensive consent decree with the FDA.

The speed of this action can be attributed to several factors, including the specter of product liability suits and the fear of general rejection of Procter & Gamble products. The FDA played an important part in the response. It was under significant public and media pressure to protect the public from TSS, despite the unanswered medical questions and the inconclusive findings in the small CDC studies. Procter & Gamble's timing was clearly determined by the FDA, who had called a meeting one day after the release of the damaging CDC study in September. The agency gave the company one week to generate evidence that the product was safe.

Despite enormous effort, Procter & Gamble could not rebut the CDC's scientific findings in that time, and it feared that overt refusal to cooperate with the FDA would have damaged the company's reputation. The result was a voluntary withdrawal of the product. This action occurred in the shadow of the FDA's powers; the decree itself states that the FDA was "contemplating the possibility of invoking the provision of [medical device law] to compel the firm" to recall Rely.[53]

ASSESSING FDA IMPACT ON
MEDICAL DEVICE INNOVATION

The goal of FDA regulation is to establish a threshold of safety and efficacy for medical devices. The regulatory process does not intend to destroy innovation or drive away "good" technology. The challenge is to establish a balance between safety and innovation. Has the balance been achieved?

Opinions are strong on all sides. Congress has generally approached the evaluation from a consumer perspective. It has sharply and regularly criticized the FDA for underregulation and failure to enforce regulatory standards. On the other hand, industry representatives have complained about unnecessary and cumbersome regulatory burdens. Who is right?

The data are inconclusive as to the effects of regulation on innovation. Generally, however, studies have indicated that, in the aggregate, device regulation has not inhibited the introduction of new goods.[54] Although few negative effects on equipment development have been found, small manufacturers may bear a greater burden than larger ones. Some researchers found that smaller firms were less likely to introduce Class III devices after device regulation was in place.[55] In a study of new product introductions of diagnostic imaging devices, however, the results offered no evidence of bias against small firms.[56]

The Medical Device Amendments of 1976 present a watershed for medical device innovators. The passage of the law forced all producers to consider the potential impact of federal regulation. This possible federal intervention, both as a barrier to and a manipulator of the marketplace, inextricably links the private producer to the FDA. The law attempted to deal with the complexity and the diversity of medical devices; it is these characteristics of the industry that have led to problems of effective regulation. Even at the lowest levels of scrutiny, compliance with FDA requirements involves time and expense to the producer. For devices in Class III, the delays and the costs are much higher.

It is obvious, however, that to firms that must meet regulatory requirements, the barriers may seem high. The impact, one can conclude, is spotty across various manufacturers and types of products. Clearly the FDA has not fully implemented all the provisions of the law, and there are powerful critics of both the FDA and the industry in Congress. If the law were fully implemented or made more stringent, then greater impacts on more firms would be inevitable. The policy question that remains, then, is whether we need more safety; if so, at what cost to the producers? Can we balance the interests of innovation and safety?[57]

Another policy designed to inhibit discovery of devices was emerging alongside the regulatory arena. Rules relating to product liability also had the potential to influence the health of our patient. It is to these legal constraints that we now turn.

6

GOVERNMENT INHIBITS
MEDICAL DEVICE DISCOVERY:
PRODUCT LIABILITY

Personal injury law allocates responsibility for the costs of accidents.[1] In product related cases, injured individuals (plaintiffs) seek to shift the costs to the producers (defendants).[2] This area of law expanded dramatically during the 1970s. The rules of liability changed so that more injured consumers had the opportunity to prevail, and the size of the awards to victorious plaintiffs tended to rise as well. The increased risk of being sued introduced new uncertainties for manufacturers and created additional potential burdens for innovators.

This increase in liability exposure occurred at the same time that medical device regulation emerged. Regulation and liability share a common goal—to deter the production of products that do not meet a standard of safety. However, these two institutions accomplish the goal in vastly different ways. Federal regulation is uniform and national. Much of the FDA's device regulation is prospective, that is, the rule is known before the manufacturer begins to market the product. (Of course, if problems arise in the marketplace, the FDA does have postmarketing surveillance power.)[3]

In contrast, liability laws vary from state to state, subjecting producers to fifty different possible sets of rules. Liability is retrospective, in that the process begins after the harm occurs. Finally, the institutions use different standards and mechanisms to determine safety. The FDA imposes primarily scientific evaluation; judges and juries apply principles rooted in law and experience rather than in science. In addition to deterrence, liability law seeks to compensate victims for the costs of the injury, leading to damage awards. Product liability also has a punitive component—the system can impose punitive damages for behavior that is particularly reprehensible.

This chapter describes the evolution of product liability law in the 1970s and the impact of those changes on medical devices. The cases of the A. H. Robins Dalkon Shield and the Pfizer-Shiley heart valve illustrate some important issues raised by liability litigation. Once again, a caveat is in order. Assessment of the impact of liability on producers is hampered by the lack of reliable data.[4] Information on settlements and litigation costs are confidential; court records are inconsistent in different states and are difficult to obtain. In addition, because of the diversity in legal requirements from state to state, generalizations about legal trends are limited. Finally, because liability rules can change with each court decision and can be altered by state or federal legislation or by voter initiative,[5] the target is a moving one. Nevertheless, trends can be identified and some conclusions can be drawn.

BREAKING LEGAL BARRIERS

Changing Theories of Liability

Until the early 1960s, there were substantial barriers to successful legal claims for injuries related to products. Several legal trends broke down those barriers so that injured individuals could more readily prevail against producers.

Negligence

To win a negligence case, the plaintiff must prove that a defendant's behavior failed to meet a legal standard of conduct and that the behavior caused the plaintiff's harm.[6] Until the midnineteenth century, negligence "was the merest dot on the law."[7] Negligence is a neutral concept, one that need not give advantage to a corporate defendant or an individual plaintiff. However, as negligence law evolved in the late nineteenth and early twentieth centuries, it supported the risk-taking behavior of industrial entrepreneurs and fit nicely within the ethic of individualism and laissez-faire.[8] Judges considered the values of economic progress; they often carefully circumscribed the defendant's duty of care and provided nearly impenetrable defenses.[9] With negligence law so limited, most cases involving product injuries relied on the rules of contract, which were quite limited in their own right.[10]

Yet, there were pressures to protect individuals injured by industrial progress. These forces increased as accidents involving railroads rose. One change in direction came in 1916, when Benjamin Cardozo, chief judge of the New York Court of Appeals, overthrew the doctrine of privity in the famous case of *MacPherson v. Buick.* A wooden automobile wheel collapsed, injuring the driver. MacPherson, the driver, sued Buick Motor Company, which had negligently failed to inspect and discover the defect. Buick's defense was that the company had no contractual relationship with MacPherson, that is, no privity of contract, because he had bought the car from a dealer, not directly from Buick. Cardozo held the manufacturer's duty of care was owed to all those who might ultimately use the product. This was a first step in the process that broke down contract law barriers placed in the way of injured persons.

A host of other doctrines, too numerous to describe here, began over the next fifty years to shift the balance in favor of the plaintiffs. By the 1960s, many state courts had greatly expanded the scope of duties owed to others, had abolished defenses available to defendants, and had begun to assess significantly higher damage awards.[11]

Product Liability

Courts began to reflect frustration with the limitations on plaintiffs under traditional contract and negligence principles. These frustrations help to explain the development of the concept of strict liability and its applicability to producers.

Strict liability (called *product liability* when applied to product cases) differs from negligence in that it is not premised on fault. The doctrine looks to the nature of the product, not the behavior of the producer. If a product is found to be defective when placed in the stream of commerce, the producer may be liable for the harm that it causes, regardless of fault. Determining the parameters of the concept of *defect* is pivotal in these cases.[12] Although strict liability had existed in the law since the nineteenth century, the theory became crucial in relation to product cases in the 1960s.

The California Supreme Court led the way when it announced the standard of strict tort liability for personal injuries caused by products in *Greenman v. Yuba Power Products*. The court held the defendant manufacturer liable for injuries caused by the defective design and construction of a home power tool. Liability was imposed irrespective of the traditional limits on warranties derived from contract law. The court stated that "[a] manufacturer is strictly liable in tort when an article he places in the market, knowing that it is to be used without inspection for defects, proves to have a defect that causes injury to a human being."[13]

Virtually every state subsequently adopted these principles of liability. Indeed, only one year after the *Greenman* case, the American Law Institute (ALI), which represents a prestigious body of legal scholars, adopted section 402A of the *Restatement (Second) of Torts*, which sets forth the strict liability standard.[14] The theory of strict liability has been elaborated and refined in various jurisdictions, including the definition of defect, the extension of the concept of defect to product design, the notion of defective warnings, and the restrictions on defenses available to the manufacturers and the duties of manufacturers when consumers misuse the product.[15]

In general, courts have held that a showing of a defect which caused[16] injury is sufficient to justify strict liability. There are three basic categories of product defects. The first is a flaw in manufacturing that causes a product to differ from the intended result of the producer. The second is a design defect that causes a product to fail to perform as safely as a consumer would expect or that creates risks that outweigh the benefits of the intended design. The third arises when a product is dangerous because it lacks adequate instructions or warnings. Cases may be brought under one or more of these categories.

Damage Awards

If a plaintiff wins the case, the next step is to assess the amount of damages to which he or she is entitled. The jury can award

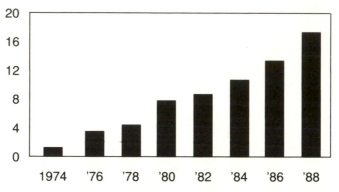

Figure 19. Product liability suits filed in federal district courts (in thousands).
Source: Administrative Office of U.S. Courts. Reprinted from *Wall Street Journal,* 22 August 1989, A16.

damages for actual out-of-pocket losses, such as medical expenses, lost wages, and property damages. In addition, juries can include noneconomic damages, such as the value of the pain and suffering of the plaintiff, a subjective judgment that can add significantly to the total award amount. The amount awarded in jury verdicts has been increasing steadily since the 1960s, and much of this increase can be attributed to medical malpractice and product liability cases.[17] (See figure 19 and table 8.)

Punitive damages are another controversial area of liability law. Theoretically, punitive damages are intended to punish wrongdoers whose conduct is particularly reprehensible. They are added on top of the award of actual damages, which are intended to fully compensate the plaintiff for losses incurred. The standards for assessing conduct are relatively vague and require few limits.[18] For many years, punitive damages played a minor role in American law. As late as 1955, the largest punitive damage verdict in the history of California was only $75,000.[19] By the 1970s, however, punitive damages were frequently awarded, with many verdicts well over one million dollars.[20]

There is considerable debate about why the liability laws changed in this way. Edward H. Levi of the University of Chicago identifies forces within the social experience of America. He believes that holding producers responsible for injuries

Table 8. Average Jury Awards in Cook County, Illinois, and San Francisco, Selected Periods, 1960–1984

Type of case	1960–64	1975–79	1980–84	Average annual percentage increase[a]		
				1960–64 to 1975–79	1975–79 to 1980–84	1960–64 to 1980–84
Medical malpractice						
Cook County	52,000	324,000	1,179,000	13.0	29.5	16.9
San Francisco	125,000	644,000	1,162,000	11.5	12.5	11.8
Product liability						
Cook County	265,000	597,000	828,000	5.6	6.8	5.9
San Francisco	99,000	308,000	1,105,000	7.9	29.1	12.8
All personal injury						
Cook County	59,000	130,000	187,000	5.4	7.5	5.9
San Francisco	66,000	133,000	302,000	4.8	17.8	7.9
Real GNP	—	—	—	3.6	2.3	3.2
Real price of medical services	—	—	—	1.9	1.1	1.7

Sources: Mark A. Peterson, *Civil Juries in the 1980s: Trends in Jury Trials and Verdicts in California and Cook County, Illinois* (Rand Corporation, Institute for Civil Justice, 1987), 22, 35, 51; and *Economic Report of the President, January 1987.*

[a]Compiled from midpoints of each five-year period.

reflects views of the 1930s, when government control was increasing generally and greater government responsibility for individual welfare was thought proper.[21] Others have argued that the change was tied to the growing complexity of products, which made consumers less able to evaluate them on an individual basis, and to the rise of the U.S. welfare state, particularly after World War II.[22] Economists Landes and Posner have an economic explanation: shifting responsibility to producers was an efficient response to urbanization and a reflection of "internalizing" costs to efficiency in manufacturing.[23] Yale law professor George Priest takes the view that modern tort law reflects a consensus of the best methods for controlling the sources of injuries related to products. Under what he calls the "theory of enterprise liability," businesses are held responsible for losses resulting from products they introduce into commerce, reflecting the perceived appropriate relationship between product manufacturers and consumers as well as the role of internalizing costs to affect accident levels and how to distribute risk.[24]

Clearly the reasons for these changes in the legal environment are complex and multiple. The extent of their impact is also controversial. Personal injury and product liability relate to all consumer products. However, pharmaceutical products have been singled out for special treatment under the law. Medical devices have not received similar consideration, although there are conflicting trends in recent court decisions.

Special Protection for Drugs, Not Devices

A special exception to strict liability has been carved out for drugs and vaccines because of their unique status in society. During debates at the American Law Institute regarding product liability, members proposed that drugs should be exempted from strict liability because it would be "against the public interest" because of the law's "very serious tendency to stifle medical research and testing." A comment (known as "comment k") following the relevant section in the *Restatement* provides that the producer of a properly manufactured prescription drug may be held liable for injuries caused by the product only if it was not accompanied by a warning of the dangers that the manufacturer knew or should have known. The comment balances basic tort law considerations of deterrence, incentives for safety, and compensation by recognizing that drugs and vaccines are unavoidably unsafe. Comment k has been adopted in virtually all jurisdictions that have considered the matter.[25]

Of course, as pharmaceutical manufacturers would be the first to say, the comment k exemption does not eliminate liability exposure. Drugs and vaccines may be exempt from design defect claims, but producers may still be held liable for failure to warn and for negligence. Because pharmaceutical products account for many of the liability actions, this exemption is quite limited in practice.[26]

Generally speaking, medical devices have been treated like all other consumer products with regard to both negligence and strict liability in most jurisdictions. A handful of cases from scattered courts, however, have grappled with the relationship of the special exemption for drugs under comment k to other medical products like medical devices. Three cases involve injuries from IUDs. While these cases do not presage any major shifts in the case law, they do provide some insight on the thorny problem of distinguishing drugs from devices in the policy-making process.

In *Terhune v. A. H. Robins*,[27] the plaintiff suffered injuries from a Dalkon Shield. She argued that A. H. Robins had failed to warn her of the risks associated with the product. The Washington State Supreme Court held that because the IUD is a prescription device, comment k applies. (The case was brought before the Medical Device Amendments had been implemented; the court said that the fact that there was no FDA approval before marketing was irrelevant.) Precedents held that the duty to warn of risks associated with prescription drugs ran only from manufacturer to physician. Prescription devices, which cannot be legally sold except to physicians, or under the prescription of a physician, are classified the same as prescription drugs for purposes of warning.

The Oklahoma Supreme Court decided a similar case several years later. In *McKee v. Moore*,[28] the plaintiff was injured by a Lippes Loop, the IUD manufactured by Ortho Pharmaceutical. As in the *Terhune* case, the plaintiff alleged that the company failed to warn of side effects. The Oklahoma Supreme Court equated prescription drugs and devices: "[U]nlike most other products, however, prescription drugs *and devices* may cause unwanted side effects even though they have been carefully and properly manufactured."[29]

The issue is somewhat different in the context of design defects. A California appellate court recently grappled with the differences between drugs and devices in the area of design. In *Collins v. Ortho Pharmaceutical*,[30] the plaintiff alleged that the Lippes Loop that injured her was defectively designed. The court, citing the *Terhune* and *McKee* cases, equated prescription drugs and prescription devices. These products have been determined to be unavoidably unsafe, said the court, because they are reviewed by the FDA and contain warnings about use. The discussion in the case seems to confuse the concept of a prescription product with the process of premarket approval. Of course, all *drugs* must undergo premarket approval by the FDA before marketing. However, as we know, the Medical Device Amendments do not require premarket screening for all devices. Indeed, the device IUDs, including the Lippes Loop, did not require PMAs when they entered the market in the early 1970s.[31] To the extent that the court is assuming that the FDA's *premarket* approval confers the unavoidably unsafe status, the analogy to devices is inapt. However, the analogy does seem appropriate for Class III devices.

Many unanswered questions remain. How much meaning does prescription confer? What about hospital equipment that is not prescribed per se, such as resuscitation equipment or monitoring apparatus? The answers are unclear, though there are important distinctions that the courts have not begun to consider.

Manufacturing defects are most frequently cited as the cause of injury in product-related suits arising from the use of medical devices. While it is increasingly common for strict liability claims to be brought in medical device cases, negligence continues to be the most common theory of recovery. The struggle in the courts on how to characterize medical devices for purposes of liability underscores the diversity of the products in the industry and the limited understanding of the relationship of devices to medical care. It also recalls the thorny drug/device distinctions that FDA and Congress grappled with in crafting regulatory principles.

The Relationship of Device Liability to Medical Malpractice

Malpractice cases are brought under negligence theory. In a medical context, the plaintiff must show that the health professional's performance fell below the standard of care in the community. The impact of medical malpractice on the practice of medicine has been the subject of much debate, which is beyond the scope of this inquiry.[32] However, there is interaction between product liability and medical practice, and that interaction has consequences for medical device producers. Fear of malpractice claims has encouraged what is known as *defensive medicine:* the practitioner is cautious, often ordering batteries of tests that may not be medically necessary in order to protect against future claims. This behavior has led to overuse of some medical technology, including medical devices.

Malpractice and product liability cases often are filed simultaneously. For example, in many IUD cases, women sue both their doctors and the product manufacturer. The manufacturer's liability is based on failure to warn of dangerous side effects or on production of a defectively designed product. A doctor's failure to inform the patient of risks associated with IUD use, failure to perform a thorough examination, negligent insertion or removal of an IUD, failure to warn of the risks of pregnancy when the device is in place, and failure to monitor the patient for adverse reactions can all establish claims.[33]

Device manufacturers have replaced physicians as the most frequently named defendants in cases involving medical device use.[34] In some instances, the physicians have allied with plaintiffs' attorneys against the manufacturer. In *Airco v. Simmons First National Bank*,[35] one of the largest medical device cases to date, the plaintiff's attorney was encouraged by the doctors whom he had charged with malpractice to sue the manufacturer of the anesthesiology equipment used in the surgery. The court held the manufacturer primarily liable for the death in the case. Airco and the physicians' partnership admitted liability for compensatory damages shortly before trial. The jury assessed $1.07 million in damages against both defendants and $3 million in punitive damages against Airco. Airco's appeal of the punitive damages award was rejected by the Arkansas Supreme Court, which found a sufficient record to support the jury's findings of a design defect in the ventilator component of Airco's breathing apparatus.

A number of states have placed caps on malpractice awards available in the courts. Legislatively imposed caps on medical malpractice may increase the likelihood that medical device manufacturers will bear additional costs to compensate injured individuals.

THE IMPACT ON DEVICE INNOVATION

There is no consensus on the size or extent of the liability crisis. Without entering that debate, it is possible to speculate on its impact on innovation in the device industry.

There is no question that the expansion of product liability has affected medical device producers. There is a greater likelihood of successful lawsuits against manufacturers and inevitably higher insurance premiums have resulted for all producers. Recently one defense attorney noted: "I'd be willing to bet that ten years ago there weren't five cases in the United States against medical device manufacturers. Now there are that many every day."[36] While data are hard to come by, this comment captures the trend. The consensus is that device producers face significant liability exposure. In general, claims are on the rise, losses have increased, and recovery rates for plaintiffs have gone up.

MEDMARC, an industry-owned insurance company for medical device manufacturers which has 440 members, may reflect the liability situation of the industry. The president of MEDMARC reported that claims rose 42 percent between 1986 and 1987. On average, the plaintiff recovery rate for hospital equipment cases is about 71 percent and for IUDs about 78 percent.[37] Many producers and service providers have experienced exceptionally high increases in insurance premiums or have been denied coverage altogether. The industries most seriously affected include manufacturers of pharmaceutical and medical devices, hospitals, physicians, and those dealing with hazardous materials.[38] For example, Puritan-Bennett, a leading manufacturer of hospital equipment such as anesthesia devices, faced a 750 percent increase in insurance premiums in 1986, with less coverage and higher deductibles.[39] Both G. D. Searle, the manufacturer of the Copper 7 IUD, and Ortho Pharmaceutical, the producer of the Lippes Loop, claim that insurance and liability exposure caused them to withdraw their product.[40]

As one might expect, the device industry asserts that innovation is threatened by this legal environment. HIMA surveyed its membership to determine its views on product liability.[41] Of the respondents, most reported soaring insurance premiums, and 25 percent reported that product liability deterred them from pursuing new products, including products that would fall into FDA Class III or that require highly skilled practitioners. Other medical organizations support this view. The American Medical Association has concluded that product liability inhibits innovative research in the development of new medical technologies.[42]

Although the data are incomplete, there is no question that the threat of product liability creates uncertainty. Except in instances of fraud or deception, producers may not know what long-term risks their products present. They may be underinsured or, in the present liability environment, unable to acquire insurance. Laws vary from state to state, laws change over time, and outcomes depend on a variety of factors unique to each case. The size of awards also varies greatly, even in instances where the actions of defendants are the same. Product liability can destroy a company or a product. However, even the most conscientious producer faces an uncertain liability future. The potential of liability policies to disrupt company operations is high. The following case studies illustrate the impact of liability laws on producers.

The Dalkon Shield

IUDs are probably the most controversial medical device in the United States. Chapter 4 discussed their entry and rapid distribution into the market in the early 1970s.[43] By the mid-1980s, the technology had practically disappeared. The story of the

Dalkon Shield has been told elsewhere in great detail.[44] It is discussed here to illustrate the impact of mass tort litigation on a firm.

Few defend the actions of A. H. Robins Company, either in the marketing of the IUD or in its subsequent behavior after the product was withdrawn. It is generally agreed that Robins entered the contraceptive market without knowledge or experience. It relied on erroneous research data, ignored warnings of product risks, and denied the existence of evidence to the contrary. The court found serious wrongdoing on the part of the company, and an official court document affirmed "a strong prima facie case that [the] defendant, with the knowledge and participation of in-house counsel, has engaged in an ongoing fraud by knowingly misrepresenting the nature, quality, safety, and efficacy of the Dalkon Shield from 1970–1984."[45]

The problem with the product has been traced to its multifilament tail, a string attached to the plastic shield (see figure 20). The string allowed women to check that the product was in place and facilitated removal by a physician. This string was not an impervious strand but was composed of many strands that allowed bacteria to be drawn from body fluids into the uterus. The result was inflammation and infection, leading to illness, sterility, and, in some instances, death.[46]

The product was removed from the market in 1974, after several deaths and 110 cases of septic abortion (miscarriage caused by infection in the uterus). Then the lawsuits began. By June 1985, there were 9,230 claims settled and 5,100 pending; Robins had paid out $378 million at that time.

The cases continued to pour in. The company filed for Chapter 11 bankruptcy protection in August 1985.[47] As part of the proceedings, a reorganization plan had to be approved, and it could not go into effect until it was clear that no legal challenges to it survived. A plan was finally approved at the end of 1989, more than four years after the initial bankruptcy filing.[48] This action cleared the way for the acquisition of the company by American Home Products and the establishment of a trust fund of $2.3 billion to compensate women who had not yet settled their claims with Robins.

The plan transferred all responsibility for the Dalkon Shield

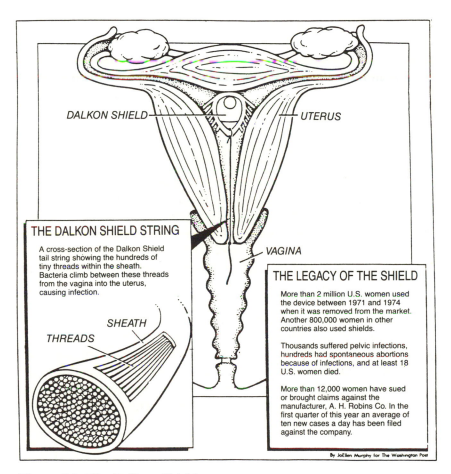

Figure 20. The Dalkon Shield.
Source: Washington Post National Weekly, 6 May 1985, 6.

claims to the trust. The trust funds were available to resolve the remaining 112,814 claims pending in 1989.[49] Twenty years after the product was marketed and sixteen years after it had been removed, injured claimants still awaited compensation. In late 1989, a federal grand jury began a criminal investigation into allegations that Robins concealed information and obstructed civil litigation.[50]

The course of this litigation raises questions about the efficiency of the tort system to accomplish its goal to compensate for injuries. It also raises issues of deterrence. Who has been deterred? Ideally, of course, only unscrupulous companies or producers of unsafe products should be deterred by liability law. However, it appears that bona fide contraception innovators have generally abandoned the market in the wake of these lawsuits. It is difficult to justify a liability system when its primary goals—compensation and deterrence—are not met.

Heart Valves

Another medical device controversy arose in 1990. This case involved the Bjork-Shiley Convexo-Concave heart valve. Heart valves regulate blood flow and are essential to an efficiently functioning heart. Defective valves can lead to constant fatigue, periodic congestive heart failure, and other ailments. The development of artificial replacement valves became a challenge to medical device producers.

In 1968, Dr. Viking O. Bjork, a Swedish professor, began working on mechanical heart valves to replace defective ones. Bjork provided the design, and the Shiley Company engineered and manufactured the valves. The design, a curved, quarter-size disk that tilted back and forth inside a metal ring, was intended to reduce the risk of blood clots, a significant problem with previous implants.[51] Approximately 394 of the 85,000 valves of this design that were sold worldwide between 1978 and 1986 have failed. The problem involves fractures in the struts that are welded on the inside of the valve that controls blood flow through the heart (see figure 21).[52] The engineering flaw that led to strut fracture in the valve caused 252 reported deaths.[53] Shiley stopped selling the valve in 1986. Over two hundred lawsuits have been filed; many more are expected.

Several tentative conclusions can be drawn from this case, although many of the legal issues were still pending in 1990. First, policy proliferation contributed to the problem. The FDA had jurisdiction over the valves. Congress began investigating the FDA's role in 1990 and accused Shiley of continuing to market the valves even after officials became aware of the manufacturing problems. Apparently as early as 1980, Shiley urged FDA officials not to notify the public because of the anxiety it

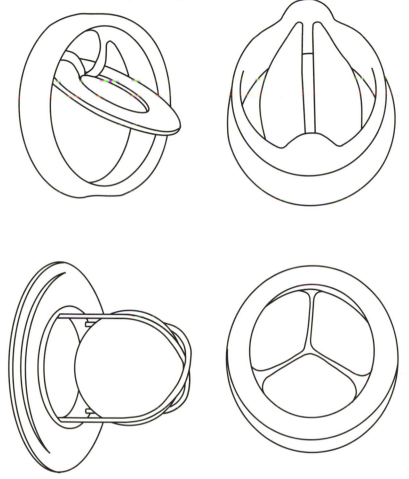

Figure 21. Examples of artificial heart valves.
Source: Marti Asner, "Artificial Valves: A Heart-Rending Story," *FDA Consumer* 15:8 (October 1981), 5.

might cause patients with implanted valves. A congressional report criticized the FDA, asserting that it was too slow in removing the valves from the market and did not properly inform the public of the risks.[54] The allegations raise important questions about the ability of the FDA to oversee the marketplace.

Another issue involves innovation. Will the legal liability facing Shiley deter others from entering the heart valve market or force current producers to withdraw from the market? Will the heart valve market soon follow the decline of the IUD industry? Will important incremental improvements in a valuable life-saving technology be lost? For example, 76,000 units of an improved Shiley monostrut (one-strut) valve have been used without failure in Europe since 1983. The FDA, claiming it needs more clinical data, has not yet approved this innovation. Is the FDA being overcautious because of the current controversy? Will this stance aggravate the deteriorating conditions for innovators?

Finally, one can ask whether litigation can resolve the dilemmas faced by patients. What about the individuals who have defective valves already implanted? They face life-threatening surgery to remove them or daily fear that the valve might fail. Does it matter that they might have died without access to the innovation in the first place? Do we have unrealistic expectations about the medical products that we use? Is the newfound anxiety legally recognizable? Some heart valve recipients have sued Pfizer on the grounds that they have increased "anxiety" knowing they are living with a defective valve. Some courts have recognized the viability of an anxiety claim, but only if Shiley engaged in fraudulent, rather than merely negligent, behavior.[55]

ASSESSING THE FATE OF TWO TECHNOLOGIES: PACEMAKERS AND IUDS COMPARED

The motivations for greater government involvement and the manner in which that involvement occurred can be illustrated by two postwar technologies—the cardiac pacemaker (see chapter 5) and the IUD. Both products had antecedents stretching back many decades, but the arrival of these modern implanted devices occurred in the 1970s and 1980s. In both cases, the products diffused rapidly and widely, so that several million women used the IUD by the mid-1970s and tens of thousands of cardiac patients had the early pacemakers implanted. There is a danger that a focus on these two technologies might skew our perceptions of the field because both generated much controversy, while thousands of other new medical devices received little or no public attention. However, comparison of these two products provides useful insights into the evolution of public policies that potentially inhibit device discovery. The public debates these devices generated led to political pressure for device regulation and illustrate the impact of the new product liability system.

It is intriguing to note that the IUD and pacemaker industries evolved quite differently by the mid-1980s. In 1986, there was only one small manufacturer of IUDs and one new entrant on the horizon. All the other major producers had withdrawn from the market, and sales were only a fraction of what they had been ten years before. The market for cardiac pacemakers, on the other hand, has continued to boom. There have been many important technological improvements. While some producers generated controversy, primarily in regard to sales tactics, early entrants prospered and many new companies thrived.

The contrast between these two innovations helps us ask important questions about the role of regulation and product liability in device innovation. The contrasts raise tantalizing questions as to why technologies succeed or fail, providing insight into the future of device innovation.

The advent of FDA regulation in the mid-1970s and the simultaneous expansion of product liability in the state courts substantially altered the interaction of the private sector and government. Inventors and developers of products could not afford either to ignore regulatory intervention before marketing a product or to ignore the regulators and the courts if subsequent risks occurred.

Regulation alone did not significantly disrupt the industry as a whole, although smaller firms bore a disproportionate share of regulatory costs. Product liability exposure presented a more general threat, particularly for evolving complex technologies, including implanted devices. The threat of liability and adverse legal outcomes work to shift costs of injuries through insurance from the consumers to the producers of products.

Pacemakers and IUDs can provide insights into the impact of these two pervasive regulatory and liability policies on innovation. There are many similarities between these two devices. Both are innovative implanted products, although the cardiac pacemaker is more complex because of its need of a power source and the need for lead wires to the heart. Both products were produced by a range of competitors for what were believed to be large markets. Both markets included large reputable firms, and innovative smaller companies. Both had unscrupulous firms. There is evidence, for example, that A. H. Robins intentionally falsified research data; Cordis Corporation has been accused of selling defective pacemakers with faulty batteries even after knowing of the defects. Four former Cordis officers have also been indicted for fraud.[56] Both technologies were subjected to significant regulation through the Class III mechanism after the law was passed. Both products gave rise to thousands of lawsuits.

Yet, by the mid-1980s, only the Alza Corporation remained in the IUD business, dominating a very small market that represented less than one-tenth the number of total sales in the IUD heyday of 1974. By contrast, the pacemaker market was booming. Medtronic, the company that pioneered the device, remained the industry leader, but many other companies maintained innovative and lucrative positions in the field.

How can we explain this disparity? What can we learn from these cases? First, the vulnerability of an innovation to adverse regulatory or product liability effects may depend on the nature of the risks the product presents. Adverse reactions to IUDs included death and sterility in young women who were otherwise healthy. Pacemakers, even if they malfunction, do not generally cause death, only a return of the symptoms.

Second, the risks presented by a product may relate not to the technology per se, but to its use by inappropriate candidates. Women for whom IUDs were inappropriate experienced severe reactions. Pacemakers implanted unnecessarily do not present greater risks than those implanted in patients who benefited from them. Also, pacemakers are used by individuals with serious preexisting medical conditions. IUDs are used by healthy young women. Adverse reactions in this population seem more unnecessary and devastating than reactions in elderly cardiac patients.

Third, both IUDs and pacemakers suffered from adverse publicity brought about by regulation and product liability cases. However, negative publicity may affect a product more if there are alternatives available for the consumers. Because there were alternatives to IUDs, it was easier for users to abandon them and switch to contraceptive pills or other barrier forms of contraception. Pacemakers continued to fulfill a critical function for which no alternative existed.

Fourth, there may be contributory effects from other public policies. The widespread availability of public Medicare funds for pacemaker implantation could have played a role in keeping the market healthy, leading to greater incremental innovation and product improvement. The market issues relevant to pacemakers will be discussed in the following chapter. The IUD did not benefit from substantial third-party payment support.

Fifth, both regulation and liability are crude tools for the prevention of product risks. Regulation attempts to operate proactively by eliminating potential risks before marketing. Arguably, this process would screen out inappropriate products, eliminating the need for product liability. Clearly the regulatory process is imperfect, because not all risks are eliminated. And the more burdensome the regulation, the more likely that desirable innovations are deterred or deflected. Product liability, a retrospective risk-reduction tool, can seriously inhibit a product or a company that produces a subsequently discovered high-risk device. Product liability may deter legitimate innovators from entering important fields of research.

It is clear that the full force of regulation and liability does not inevitably eliminate innovations. The pacemaker has remained a viable product, even in the face of controversy, and incremental innovative improvements have been continuously produced. Although the IUD did not flourish, the technology remains viable. Indeed, the efforts of two small companies, Alza Corporation and GynoPharma, which are discussed in Chapter 7, illustrate how firms can adapt controversial technologies to the current regulatory and liability environment.

Indeed, as policies have proliferated, their effects on the industry can only be understood in relationship to one another. It seems clear that the introduction of policies to inhibit device discovery—regulation and product liability—have negative effects on some products. However, the whole free-spending environment generated by government payment policies tended

to blunt the impact of regulation and liability. This environment, however, began to change when cost control became the
theme of the 1980s. When efforts to inhibit device distribution
began in earnest, the potential for serious impacts on innovators
emerged.

7

GOVERNMENT INHIBITS MEDICAL DEVICE DISTRIBUTION

	Discovery	Distribution
Promote	1. National Institutes of Health (NIH) Space & Defense Spinoffs	2. Hill-Burton Hospital Construction Funds Medicare/Medicaid
Inhibit	3. Regulation (FDA) Product Liability	4. Certificate of Need Cost-Containment Technology Assessment

Figure 22. The policy matrix.

The federal and state payment programs described in chapter 4 provided little incentive for hospitals, providers, or eligible patients to consider costs when making decisions about health care. As a result, there were few economic barriers to the use of any new and apparently safe technology. Even the advent of regulation and the expansion of product liability in the 1970s did not appear to slow the growth of the health care technology market, at least in the aggregate.

However, concerns about the escalating costs of health care generated new attitudes toward medical delivery systems. The belief that more is better gave way to assertions that the system was too large, unwieldy, and wasteful. From the early 1970s through the mid-1980s, at least one dozen major federal laws were enacted in response to spiraling medical costs.[1] The dominant statutory and regulatory theme was cost containment. These new laws did not constitute revolutionary change. They did presage a conceptual shift, however, toward two potentially conflicting goals—promotion of competition in health care and greater government regulation and control.[2]

This chapter reviews the impact of government cost-control measures on the distribution of medical devices. Many considered medical technology a key culprit in the rising costs of health care. One widely cited 1979 study estimated that the contribution of new technology to hospital cost increases ran as high as 50 percent.[3] There is no question that the cost-containment policies intended to slow the introduction and the diffusion of new technologies, particularly cost-raising products. The justification was that effective controls would not only reduce costs but also improve care because unconstrained diffusion led to excessive tests, treatments, and risks as well. (See figure 22.)

There are three types of cost-containment strategies: behavioral, budgetary, and informational. Behavioral regulation tries to inhibit diffusion by modifying the behavior of medical decision makers. These policies influence decisions about use, expansion, and acquisition of technology. Prime examples of this policy strategy are the state based certificate-of-need programs (CON), described in more detail below. Budgetary regulation sets rates or expenditures, leaving administrators free to manage within the cost constraints established by the payers. Budgetary controls are epitomized by Medicare's prospective payment system (PPS). Informational regulation inhibits the adoption and diffusion of new medical technologies through prospective evaluation techniques, including technology assessment and the newer outcomes, or effectiveness, research.

Case studies illustrating the potentially powerful impact of these policies on the adoption and diffusion of medical devices include the intraocular lens (IOLs), artificial replacement lenses implanted after cataract surgery, and cochlear implants, permanently implanted devices that mitigate severe hearing impairment. Both of these cases demonstrate the impact of payment policies on the introduction of new devices. Also, they highlight the collective impact of a broad range of policies—from NIH, to

FDA, to HCFA—on the entire innovation process. By the 1970s and 1980s, policy proliferation was in full swing.

POLICY OVERVIEW
Regulation of Market Behavior

The early cost-containment programs of the 1970s have been characterized as behavioral in that they tried to block decisions by providers about use, expansion, and acquisition of technology.[4] The goal was to eliminate waste and unnecessary expenditure, in order to save the cost-based reimbursement system.

One such effort was Title XVI of the National Health Planning and Resources Development Act of 1974, which supplanted the Hill-Burton program.[5] These new controls stipulated that federal subsidies to eligible institutions must be made in compliance with statewide cost-control plans. In the 1970s, government subsidies became less important than other sources of funds, and the influence of these controls diminished considerably.

In 1972, Congress also authorized establishment of federally funded, private Professional Standards Review Organizations (PSROs) to conduct independent quality and utilization reviews of hospital services under Medicare and Medicaid.[6] These efforts were highly controversial. Congress formally terminated the program ten years later, replacing it with an alternative peer-review approach. The Professional Review Organizations (PROs) established under the 1983 Medicare reform, discussed below, intended to monitor hospitals to determine if Medicare payments were appropriate.

The statewide plans referred to in the health planning legislation generally meant certificate-of-need programs. New York state's passage of a certificate-of-need law in 1964 was the first government sponsored investment control. Concern about the inflation in health care costs led to the rapid diffusion of these types of controls. By 1978, thirty-eight states had adopted similar programs. State programs varied widely in terms of the types of institutions covered by the controls, thresholds for review, and legal sanctions for failure to comply.[7]

The goals of these laws generally were to eliminate "unnecessary" expansion of hospitals and to encourage less costly alternatives to hospital care. The easiest measure of these goals was excess bed capacity. Certificate-of-need agencies were predisposed to disapprove a hospital's proposal for new beds and spent considerable time and energy reviewing them. However, it is argued that controls were less successful when reviewing new services and equipment proposals, for several reasons: the costs of acquiring information about services and equipment are high, denials open the agency to charges of withholding from citizens the benefits of medical progress, and denials are likely to raise the ire of physician groups who want access to the same equipment that their colleagues have at other hospitals.[8] The evidence indicates that certificate-of-need programs resulted in no significant effect on total investments among hospitals but did alter the composition of those investments. Specifically, there was lower growth of bed supplies and higher growth of plant assets per bed. Thus, for most areas of medical device technology, these particular cost-containment strategies probably had little or no impact.

Regulation through Budgetary Constraints

An alternative means to control hospital inputs is to put caps on reimbursements paid to hospitals from the federal and state governments. In September 1982, Congress directed the Department of Health and Human Services (HHS) to propose a plan to revise the Medicare payment system. That December, the Health Care Financing Administration (HCFA), the agency responsible for processing Medicare claims, proposed a prospective payment plan. Medicare had been building empirical data on this type of reimbursement scheme with demonstration projects in several states. Congress passed the Social Security Amendments of 1983 the following March, with most of the new provisions to be gradually phased in over a three-year period.[9]

In brief, the plan created a complex prospective payment system, known as PPS. Medicare now bases its prices for Medicare hospital cases on a comprehensive classification system comprised of about 470 mutually exclusive categories called "diagnostic related groups" (DRGs). The basic assumption is that all illnesses can be grouped according to disease system, intensity of resources consumed, and length of stay, among other categories, and that such groups reflect the average cost of providing services to all patients with diseases in that DRG. The price is then determined by calculating an average price per case for all Medicare cases plus the weight of the DRG assigned to the particular patient's case. The hospital is reimbursed at a price set in advance for each DRG rather than the actual cost of treatment. As of 1988, DRG reimbursement applied only to inpatient care. Physicians' services continued to be paid out on the old "reasonable cost" basis, but Congress passed legislation to extend a form of prospective payment to physicians in the 1990s.[10]

Congress understood that the prospective rate-setting process needed the flexibility to respond to advances in all health care technology. Congress created the Prospective Payment Assessment Commission (ProPAC) to participate in the process of updating the hospital payment rates in an independent and public fashion. ProPAC members are appointed by the Office of Technology Assessment (OTA), which is a congressional advisory body, and ProPAC's seventeen members must represent a wide range of constituencies. Its responsibilities under the law are to make annual recommendations to HHS on the appropriate percentage change in Medicare payments for hospital services and to make recommendations on necessary changes in the DRGs, including the establishment of new groups, modification of existing groups, and changing their relative weights when appropriate. HHS is not bound to adopt the recommendations of ProPAC and, to date, has not done so in many cases.[11]

The intended effect of this dramatically new payment structure was to encourage efficient delivery of health care services in the hospital sector, ultimately reducing federal Medicare expenditures. The intention to stabilize or reduce the market size as well as to inhibit unnecessary expenditures on underutilized equipment was an important goal. Consistent reductions in aggregate equipment expenditures have not, apparently, occurred, although sales in some SIC categories leveled off for a time because of uncertainty about the future.

The true impact of the new program on medical device producers has been mitigated somewhat because it has not been fully implemented. At the end of the 1980s, one major issue relating to medical equipment had not been resolved. Congress deferred a decision on how the system should treat major capital expenditures by hospitals. Many medical devices, such as diagnostic equipment and monitoring and anesthesia products, fall into this category.

Under the cost-plus system of reimbursement before PPS, hospitals prepared capital-cost reports for Medicare. Medicare paid 100 percent of the reasonable costs of capital equipment (defined as land, buildings, and movable equipment) that were attributed to the care of Medicare patients in each hospital cost center. This procedure was known as the *capital-cost pass-through*, and it provided incentives for hospitals to expand and improve their capital base. The payment program, along with the growth of private insurance that provided stable cash flow, improved the borrowing power of hospitals and encouraged them to finance construction and equipment acquisition through debt. Hospital capital pass-throughs accounted for about 8 percent of the total Medicare spending in fiscal 1984 (with 14 percent of that attributable to depreciation of movable assets—that is, devices), a modest but important aspect of the financial picture for hospitals.[12]

When PPS passed in 1983, Congress initially excluded capital-related costs from the prospective payment system, deferring a decision on the issue until October 1986. At the time, Congress sought more information because of the complexity of hospital capital spending and because of the variations in investment cycles that might give arbitrary advantages to hospitals with recently completed capital expansion if controls were imposed on a specific date.[13]

Congress proposed several capital-cost plans in 1985, but voted in 1986 and 1987 simply to reduce the percentage of capital-cost pass-through payments (phased in from a 3.5 percent reduction in 1987 to a 15 percent reduction in 1988), without tackling the more difficult task of folding capital costs into the prospective payment system. These congressional efforts prevented HCFA from imposing its own rules.[14]

By the end of the 1980s, then, there was a two-tiered payment system for equipment, allowing pass-throughs for capital but controlling all other hospital expenditures. The system has benefited equipment producers, at least in the short run. The expectation was that if costs for labor and services were controlled and capital equipment costs could be passed through, then hospitals would channel funds into capital projects and the purchase of labor-saving equipment. Indeed, a 1988 study found that spending for major movable equipment, in particular, increased after 1983.[15]

Debates on how to finally structure capital costs continued through the 1980s. HCFA urged merging capital costs into PPS. ProPAC, however, changed course in 1990 and opposed any change in the capital-cost program. Capital spending continued to rise, jumping 28 percent in 1989 to $15 billion. HCFA approved one-third of that amount, or about $5 billion in Medicare capital spending. This amount represented about 9 percent of the program's $58 billion, part A budget. Estimates for 1990 were $19.3 billion, up another 27 percent.[16]

PPS could have had a much greater impact on innovative medical technology if the original plan had been fully implemented. Through the 1980s, the capital-cost pass-through operated as a modest safety valve on some innovative devices that are considered capital equipment. Yet, continuation of the debate into the 1990s underscores the pervasive market uncertainty facing medical device producers.

Information through Technology Assessment

Another technique to control the adoption and diffusion of technology is to assess it prospectively. If a new technology does not pass the evaluation screen, a market barrier can be imposed. Ongoing comparative assessment can promote the abandonment of outdated technologies and thereby affect the rate of diffusion.

Prospective assessment is not limited to evaluation on the basis of cost. Indeed, the concept, as originally conceived, was quite broad. The idea was formally developed by Congressman Emilio Daddario, chair of the House Subcommittee on Science, Research, and Development in 1965.[17] His work recognized that scientific and technological developments present potential social consequences. The goal of technology assessment was to examine the safety, efficacy, indications for use, cost, and cost-effectiveness of a particular technology, including the social, economic, and ethical consequences to improve health care decisions.[18]

While the concept of medical technology assessment sounds high-minded, its implementation raised a number of very complex issues. Assessment involves three levels of information: gathering of data, evaluating data, and imposing decisions through regulation based upon the evaluation. In addition, assessments can apply to a broad range of technologies—drugs, devices, procedures, and systems—or to just one. Finally, assessment can cover many attributes of a technology, including safety or cost, or it can be limited to only one attribute. Thus, for example, the Food and Drug Administration can be considered a technology assessment agency. Its jurisdiction extends to drugs and devices (not procedures); it evaluates the attributes of safety and efficacy only (not cost or cost-effectiveness); it can require data gathering from the producer; and it regulates based on its evaluation of the data.

It is clear that those who control technology assessments become pivotal gatekeepers for adoption and diffusion of that technology. Thus the history of medical technology assessment is inextricably linked to the tensions among interest groups to influence assessment results. Much of the battle has also involved private sector efforts to prevent government from increasing its share of the gatekeeper function. This concern is especially acute when the goals of the government are to contain costs and arguably to prevent innovations from entering the marketplace, particularly if they are perceived to increase costs.

Government agencies entered the technology assessment process at an early stage to accomplish a variety of goals. As might be expected, government efforts were piecemeal and underfunded. The market does not generate necessary and complete information on medical technologies because clinical testing is time-consuming and expensive. It is easy for competitors to become free riders by observing the technological choices of others. Government plunged ahead. In addition to the FDA, new programs were created in both the administrative and the legislative branches of government, including the Health Program at the Office of Technology Assessment (legislative branch), the National Center for Health Services Research (NCHSR), the NIH's Office of Medical Applications of Research (OMAR), and, for a short time, the National Center for Health Care Technology (NCHCT). HCFA uses the services of the Offices of Health Technology Assessment (OHTA) within HHS to provide assessment data. OHTA has a very small budget and is limited to safety and efficacy review.[19]

Both producer and physician groups in the private sector resented government efforts to control technology. Their opposition has been particularly intense when a government agency has the power to regulate decision making rather than the ability just to gather information. For example, in 1978 the American Medical Association (AMA) opposed the creation of the NCHCT, which had regulatory power, alleging that it would interfere with medical practice. HIMA argued that the new assessment agency was a threat to innovation. Both groups strongly and successfully advocated the dismantling of the agency in 1982.[20]

When PPS passed, cost control became an important federal goal. Despite their concerns, technology producers understood that information about benefits as well as costs was now essential for government. A cost-conscious government payer (HCFA) accounted for the direct and the indirect purchasers of over 40 percent of all medical technology. HCFA would gather information regardless of whether the industry or professions cooperated. Government clearly assumed an important and indisputable role. Indeed, as the 1980s progressed, cost dominated the technology assessment debate, and HCFA established itself in a leadership position. Many private payers followed its lead.

Many believed, although HCFA vehemently denied it, that the agency made coverage decisions based predominantly on cost issues, at least since the inception of PPS. The debate about HCFA's jurisdiction and authority to evaluate a technology's cost-effectiveness in order to make coverage determinations illustrates the nature of the debate.

The legislative mandate of HCFA is to decide whether a medical service is "reasonable and necessary" in order to provide Medicare coverage. Many coverage decisions are made by insurers that contract with Medicare, and there is much regional variation. However, some major coverage decisions are made by the national agency.[21] In a rule proposed in 1989, HCFA attempted to clarify the meaning of "reasonable and necessary" under the Medicare program. It proposed to add the criterion of cost-effectiveness to considerations of safety and effectiveness; it also proposed to consider whether a technology was experimental or investigational. It justified its proposal thus: "HCFA is including cost-effectiveness as a criterion because we believe considerations of cost are relevant in deciding whether to expand or continue coverage of technologies, particularly in the context of the current explosion of high-cost technologies."[22]

Both the AMA and HIMA opposed the addition of cost-effectiveness as a coverage criterion, arguing that it raised substantial legal, methodological, and policy questions. The AMA also argued that HCFA lacked the statutory authority to make the decision and that Medicare's purpose is to meet medical needs, not to make evaluations and comparisons among technologies that amount to the practice of medicine. It also argued that cost-effectiveness analysis is impractical, time-consuming, and inherently subjective.[23] HIMA had similar concerns, and added that cost should be a factor only in reimbursement decisions, not for coverage policy. HIMA stated that the proposal would provide a major barrier to entry for new technology. These concerns of organized medicine and industry echo their complaints against the now-defunct NCHCT. No action had been taken on the proposal by 1990. Regardless of the outcome, however, it is likely that HCFA will take cost into consideration, either overtly with clarified authority or somewhat more indirectly.

Cost-effectiveness considerations have also crept into other technology assessments. A recent example involves the deliberations of the FDA Advisory Panel on Obstetrics and Gynecology Devices. The FDA has no statutory authority to consider costs in its deliberations; it is limited by law to considerations of safety and efficacy. However, the advisory panel voted unanimously against approval of Healthdyne's home uterine monitoring systems for premature labor.[24] The device reads the uterine activity of a pregnant woman and transmits it by modem to a professional in a clinical setting. The advisory panel was concerned about the absence of direct clinical proof that product use reduced morbidity or mortality, although others argued that in vitro diagnostics have never been required to produce such data. Also apparent in the advisory panel deliberations were concerns that the technology would become a costly new standard of care. The American College of Obstetricians and Gynecologists (ACOG) issued a statement that the device would cost about $80 a day, averaging $5,616 per patient and potentially costing $5.6 billion a year. Observers commented that costs appeared to have influenced the panel's decision to disapprove the device: "FDA advisory panels are intended to guide the agency on product safety and efficacy and risk-benefit. Increasingly, especially in the area of devices, panels have come under pressure from . . . [HCFA] . . . to factor in cost-benefit considerations as well."[25]

The trend for the 1990s is movement from traditional technology assessment to the measurement of outcomes. Broadly conceived, outcomes research measures the patient's quality of life as the result of medical treatment. Purchasers are seeking value for their money, and providers are interested in how to ensure the best quality care. While the thrust of outcomes research is slightly different from technology assessment, the barriers to its attainment are similar. There is no consensus on how to measure outcomes or who should pay for it.

Despite these problems, Congress demonstrated its support for the concept of outcomes research with the 1989 creation of the Agency for Health Care Policy and Research (AHCPR) to "enhance the quality, appropriateness, and effectiveness of health care services and to improve access to services."[26] Congress appropriated $568 million over the next five years to fund its activities. Among its goals are the facilitation of practice guidelines to assist physicians, a treatment effectiveness program to assess the effects of variations of treatment on outcomes, and support for programs in health services research and training of researchers.

Many express optimism about the potential for outcomes research. But even in its earliest stages, there is mutual distrust between payers and providers and a belief that payers will assess technology on the basis of cost, not quality. As one observer put it, "[W]hat looks like effectiveness research from one perspective looks like cost-cutting from another. Providers continue to distrust the long reach of government; government looks with narrowed eyes on the amount spent for providers' services."[27]

CASE STUDIES: THE IMPACT OF GOVERNMENT COST CONTAINMENT ON DISTRIBUTION

The introduction of cost containment into government payment policies has had and will continue to have a powerful impact on medical device producers. HCFA is now as important a barrier as the FDA. Medicare coverage and payment policies can delay and limit access of an innovation to the marketplace. Most importantly, market access becomes problematical. There are no clear policy guidelines for producers as HCFA continually experiments with regulatory approaches, and Congress periodically intervenes as a watchdog and accomplice in the search for ways to control government spending. Additionally, there are short-run market distortions based on the idiosyncrasies of the Medicare system. For example, imposing DRGs on the hospitals only opened opportunities in the less regulated outpatient segment of Medicare. How long that differential will last is not known, as extensions of PPS to physicians' fees and outpatient settings were on the horizon in 1990. Once again, the future is uncertain, hampering long-term strategic planning in the industry.

The following case studies illustrate the powerful influence of government payment policies on a new technology. They also introduce the realities of policy proliferation. Cost containment appeared in an already complex, regulated market. In the cases of the intraocular lens and the cochlear implant, the interrelationships of the multiple policies play a role in the potential success or failure of the technologies.

Intraocular Lenses

Millions of Americans suffer from eye diseases that impair vision. Cataracts, opacities of the lens of the eye, often result from degenerative changes in old age or from diseases such as diabetes. The symptoms include gradual loss of vision, and treatment most commonly involves removal of the diseased lens and the implantation of an intraocular lens (IOL) to restore sight.[28]

Ophthalmology in general, and IOLs in particular, represent one of the largest and most dynamic health care markets. The FDA regulates IOLs, and, because most of the implant candidates are elderly, the market is strongly tied to Medicare payment policy. This policy, as well as the interaction between regulation and reimbursement, has the potential for significant impact on the industry.

IOLs are one of the few ophthalmic products that the FDA has placed in Class III.[29] Regulated since 1979, IOLs are subject to a special requirement imposed by Congress and enforced by the FDA.[30] As with all Class III devices, the FDA reviews data on safety and efficacy in the premarket approval (PMA) application. During the experimental stage, Class III products may receive an IDE, or investigational device exemption, that allows them to be used in controlled studies while the manufacturer gathers and evaluates the data about their safety and efficacy. The collection of data supporting a PMA is expensive and time-consuming and may represent a significant barrier to entry for smaller innovative firms. For IOLs, however, a special exception was made whereby the producers could charge for the costs of the implanted lenses while still in the investigational (IDE) stage. This exemption facilitated the development of IOLs during the two or more years of FDA-required device testing in clinical settings.

Indeed, the availability of Medicare payment for this primarily elderly patient population essentially guaranteed a large, stable market for lens removal and IOL implantation. The average cataract patient is sixty-eight years old; Medicare is the sole payer for almost all cataract surgery. The frequency of IOL implants has grown rapidly in the 1980s. In 1979, there were 177,000 implants; by 1986, the number was 888,000. By 1988, there were 1.2 million implants in the United States and another one million internationally. Annual IOL sales have been estimated at $360 million in the United States alone (see table 9).[31]

Medicare pays close to $1.5 billion annually for cataract oper-

Table 9. 1988 Intraocular Lens Market

	U.S.	Abroad	Total/Average
Number of cataract procedures (in millions)	1.2	2.4	3.6
Number of IOL implants (in millions), including secondary implants	1.2	1.0	2.2
Average unit price	$300	$240	$275
Use of specialty lenses	85%	60%	75%
Procedure growth rate/year (through 1990)	7%	18%	13%
Market size ($ millions)	$360	$240	$600

Source: Biomedical Business International 12:5 (16 May 1989): 70.

ations, making them the largest item in the Medicare program in 1988.[32] During the 1980s much of the treatment shifted from hospital to outpatient surgery centers or physicians' offices, which are covered under Part B of Medicare and thus are not under the DRG system. The growth can be attributed to advances in the technology, including cataract management, anesthesia, surgical technique, and postoperative care. New IOL technology includes soft lenses that can be implanted with smaller incisions (the one-stitch lens is a recent innovation), and bifocal implants and other specialty lenses have been developed recently.

The industry is dynamic and competitive. There are a number of companies in the IOL field, ranging from very large firms such as Johnson & Johnson (IOLAB), CooperVision (recently acquired by Alcon/Nestle), and Allergan (purchased by Smith-Kline Beecham in 1989). Smaller firms include IOPTEX Research, a privately held industry leader, and Chiron Ophthalmics, a subsidiary of Chiron Corporation, a biotechnology firm. There are also foreign IOL makers from West Germany, France, Belgium, Israel, and Japan.

Changes in both Medicare policy and FDA regulations present threats to the IOL market. Congress has reduced federal

Medicare payments for cataract surgery twice since 1986. HCFA has lowered the amount of payment to physicians for the procedure. These changes have come in the wake of allegations of market abuse by cataract surgeons. Congress investigated the situation as early as 1985;[33] additional hearings were held in 1990, prompted by reports that surgeons employed abusive marketing techniques to round up elderly patients, and that many earned more than $1 million a year performing surgery covered by Medicare.[34]

In 1990, HCFA reduced the payment rate for an IOL implanted during cataract extraction. The revised rate of $200 meant an average reduction of at least $100 from the former IOL rate.[35] This lower rate was based on an audit by the Office of the Inspector General to determine how much was actually paid for lenses after subtracting various rebates and discounts often associated with lens purchases. However, many of the newer specialty lenses average over $300 each.

The FDA has imposed new requirements for data collection as well. For new bifocal and multifocal products, fifty implants have to be studied for a year, and then the studies can be expanded to five hundred implants. Overall, it is likely to take nearly four years for a new lens to receive premarket approval. The longer period for approval is less onerous if the innovator receives at least partial payment for the experimental lens implants. Rumors have been circulating that the exemption allowing payment for IOLs under IDEs will soon be rescinded. HCFA officials state that this move will encourage producers to progress from the IDE to the PMA stage. They assert that companies have been allowing products to languish under IDEs because the economic incentive to go to market is reduced by the exception. The device is paid for in either case. However, the longer testing requirements and the threatened withdrawal of payment during the investigational period potentially will have a significant impact on newer, less well-capitalized entrants.

Cochlear Implants

Cochlear implants, a technology that permits individuals with profound hearing loss to receive auditory cues, have had a very different reception than IOLs. Unlike implanted lenses that diffused rapidly to millions of elderly, cochlear implants have not fared well. Indeed, Medicare reimbursement was made for only sixty-nine such implants in fiscal 1987, despite estimates that sixty thousand to two hundred thousand Americans could benefit from the device. Many industrial competitors never entered the field or have since abandoned it, leaving only three firms still in the market in 1990. This medical device has met resistance throughout its history, and the collective impact of policy hurdles has been profound.

The cochlea, a structure in the inner ear, translates sounds from mechanical vibrations to electrical signals. These signals are produced by cells in the cochlea. The cells have a fringe of tiny hairs that bend in response to vibrations in the outer and middle ear. Those responses produce electrical signals that stimulate the auditory nerve and send messages that the brain interprets as sound.[36]

This natural system of hearing is versatile enough to transmit the full range of sounds. If the hair cells in the cochlea are damaged by injury or disease, the individual is condemned to deafness. Over two hundred thousand Americans suffer this profound hearing loss, and conventional hearing aids are useless for them. Cochlear implants, at least at this stage of development, cannot restore the world of sound. They do allow for reception of sounds such as sirens and voices, auditory cues that are vital for safety and for some social interactions. But the recipient of the implant cannot hear normal conversation.

The possibility of producing useful hearing by electrical stimulation of the cochlea occurred by accident.[37] When an amplifier used in the operating room to monitor the cochlear response oscillated, the patient heard a very high-pitched tone. Some early work on this type of induced stimulation was published in 1955 and 1956.[38] Researchers undertook additional work during the early 1960s, but they encountered significant problems. Among the barriers were included adverse patient reactions to the insulating silicone rubber used in the first primitive devices and concern about the effects of long-term stimulation on all auditory sensation. In 1965, the results of studies were submitted to the American Otological Society but were rejected as too controversial for presentation.

As implant technology improved in the late 1960s, some of the problems were resolved, but concerns over ethics and long-term effects still dogged the technology. The National Institutes of Health did not provide any funding for the scientific research, a refusal that some scientists in the field attributed to the bias against biomedical engineering among NIH peer review groups.[39]

Several policy breakthroughs occurred in the 1970s, when the NIH focus began to shift toward goal oriented, or targeted, programs that would produce identifiable results. The NIH established an intramural program to investigate cortical and sub-cortical stimulation, primarily for blindness but also for other neurological disorders. While hearing stimulation was not an important part of the original program, it became of greater interest when the research on cortical visual implants appeared clearly unsuccessful. In 1977, the NIH instituted an independent assessment of patients with cochlear implants. The Bilger Report, produced at the University of Pittsburgh, concluded that these products were a definite aid to communication.[40]

Seven years later, in November 1984, the FDA approved the design of a single-channel device for cochlear implantation. The 3M Company produced the device in conjunction with Dr. William House, an early researcher and chief inventor. The device consisted of a receiver similar to that of a hearing aid, a speech-processing minicomputer that transforms the sound signals into electrical signals, another receiver for those electrical signals that is implanted under the skin above and behind the ear, and a thin wire inserted surgically through the mastoid bone into the cochlea to transmit the signals (see figure 23).

By 1985 a handful of companies had entered the market. The 3M Company was the clear leader with the only approved product. Others included the Nucleus Group, an Australian company and parent of the U.S. Cochlear Corporation, Biostim, and Symbion, an outgrowth of research at the University of Utah.[41] A private industry group reported that leading hearing-aid manufacturers did not enter the marketplace because "the FDA-

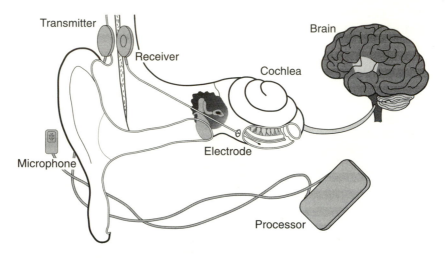

Figure 23. The cochlear implant.
Source: The 3M Company, Cochlear Implant System, n.d.

related expense of developing and testing such devices is pro-
hibitive." It was reported that 3M had budgeted over $15 million
for cochlear implant development.

Once approved by the FDA, the device faced the hurdle of
Medicare's coverage and payment decision. After several years
of deliberation, and following endorsement of the device by the
AMA in 1983 and the American Academy of Otolaryngology in
1985, Medicare issued a favorable coverage ruling for both
single-channel and multichannel devices in September 1986.
The next step was for HCFA to assign the technology to a code
which would then provide the means for establishing appropriate levels of payment for procedures.[42]

HCFA has considerable discretion in the placement of a new
procedure into the DRG system. If the device is assigned to a
DRG that does not cover the cost during the diffusion period,
hospitals implanting the devices will lose money. Hospitals that
increase the proportion of cases involving these devices lower
their operating margins in those DRGs. ProPAC recommended
in 1987 that the cochlear implant be assigned to a device specific,
temporary DRG. HCFA did not follow ProPAC's recommendation. Instead, in May 1988 the agency announced a DRG place-

ment that would not pay the full estimated cost of $14,000 for the implantation of the device.[43]

Evidence accumulated that hospitals had a strong disincentive to provide cochlear implantation. Ten percent of the 170 hospitals involved openly acknowledged to researchers that they restricted implantations because of the loss of $3,000 to $5,000 for each Medicare case.[44]

These policies limited the size of the market and deeply affected the private sector producers. The 3M Company stopped marketing the single-channel model actively and halted research on multichannel devices because of the low use rate of both models. The small market discouraged additional investment. There were five firms that developed cochlear implants for the U.S. market from 1978 through 1985. By 1990, three had left and there were no new entrants with FDA approved devices.[45]

It was undisputed that this new technology had limitations, but it also was recognized as useful and beneficial to certain classes of patients. The policy environment was relatively unresponsive to early development. The quest for FDA approval was difficult, time-consuming, and costly. The response of HCFA to the technology was definitely obstructionist. The future of the research and development of this area of technology is now in doubt.

The primary effect of the payment policy has been uncertainty in the marketplace. Firms can no longer count upon growth in their particular market segment. Incremental policy changes are frequent and can have catastrophic effects on the markets for some products. In addition, cost-containment policies have introduced new hurdles to market access, which cause higher costs and delays even for successful new entrants.

Cost control has become an important value in the distribution of medical devices. It presents significant problems because the costs of a new technology are difficult to predict before distribution. Some products may have cost-reducing potential that is not known in the early stages or additional beneficial applications that will emerge during use. It is legitimate to ask how much cost should matter and who should decide that issue.

In addition, the case studies illustrate how complex the policy environment was in 1990. There are significant hurdles at virtually every stage of innovation. Even promoters such as NIH can place barriers in the paths of the innovators. NIH disapproval can act as a deterrent, as the early years of cochlear implant development reveal. HCFA, once a source of nearly unlimited funds, can significantly delay or even bar technology from the marketplace.

Our medical device patient is now a confirmed recipient of polypharmacy, as the prescriptions have proliferated over time. Before we turn to the prognosis, however, it is necessary to look at the international marketplace. Does the world market provide an outlet for manufacturers constrained by cost controls in the United States? Or are international firms a competitive threat both in the United States and abroad?

8

THE INTERNATIONAL MARKETPLACE: SAFETY VALVE OR COMPETITIVE THREAT?

By the end of the 1980s, the United States medical device market was fraught with uncertainties, particularly as cost-containment pressures grew. International sales opportunities offered a safety valve for American device producers. Foreign competitors, on the other hand, tried to dominate the markets both in their own countries and in the United States.

This chapter provides an overview of the international medical device market. American device firms must compete in an increasingly international marketplace. Penetration of these markets depends on not only trade and tariff issues but also an understanding of government policies on health care regulation and delivery. Three case studies illustrate specific international challenges. The discussion shows how regulation and the structure of health care delivery in Japan affect foreign producers; how efforts at harmonization dominate European concerns; and how China represents the challenges of international competitors in a large and developing marketplace.

OVERVIEW OF THE INTERNATIONAL MARKET

Throughout the 1980s, the United States dominated the $36.1 billion worldwide market for medical devices and equipment. America produced 62.3 percent of the world market share and consumed 59.3 percent, or over $20 billion in sales. Japan was a distant second, producing nearly 16 percent of medical equipment consumed worldwide and spending 12.3 percent, or $5 billion annually. West Germany ranked third, with 9.1 percent production and 6.9 percent consumption. Other western Euro-

179

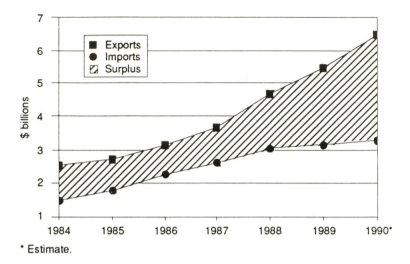

* Estimate.

Figure 24. United States exports and imports of health care technology products, 1984–1990.

Source: U.S. Department of Commerce. Reprinted from Health Industry Manufacturers Association, *Competitiveness of the U.S. Health Care Technology Industry* (1991), 13.

pean countries consumed 9.5 percent and produced 6.7 percent, and all other countries combined accounted for only 6 percent production and 12 percent consumption.[1]

Despite these positive statistics, there are mixed signals for U.S. medical device producers. The favorable balance of U.S. trade worldwide has been sliding since 1981. The trend was downward from 1983 to 1987 (see figures 24–27). The slight improvement in 1987 has been generally attributed to the favorable U.S. exchange rates.[2] Department of Commerce data show that for medical device products between 1983 and 1987 the average annual growth rate for exports was 8.9 percent, while imports were more than twice that at 20.4 percent.

The trade balance with Japan shows a more precipitous decline for the United States, with a fall to a trade deficit in 1984 (see figure 28). This deficit occurred because exports to Japan did not rise as fast as did imports of Japanese medical device products to America. American and Japanese consumption and trade patterns since 1968 are shown in table 10.

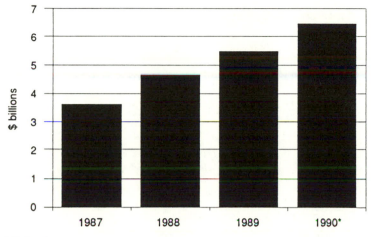

* Estimate.

Figure 25. United States medical products exports, 1987–90.
Source: U.S. Department of Commerce. Reprinted from Health Industry Manufacturers Association, *Competitiveness of the U.S. Health Care Technology Industry* (1991), 13.

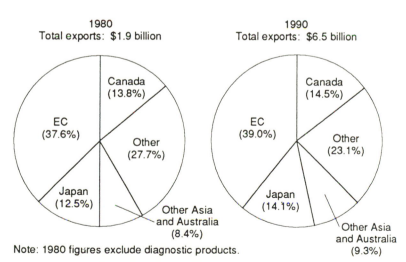

Note: 1980 figures exclude diagnostic products.

Figure 26. Major purchasers of United States medical products exports, 1980 and 1990.
Source: U.S. Department of Commerce. Reprinted from Health Industry Manufacturers Association, *Competitiveness of the U.S. Health Care Technology Industry* (1991), 15.

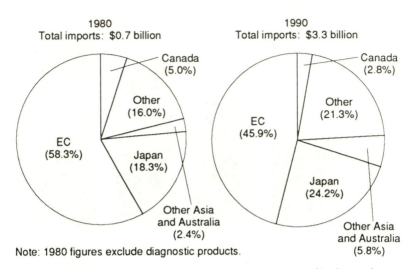

1980
Total imports: $0.7 billion

Canada
(5.0%)

Other
(16.0%)

EC
(58.3%)

Japan
(18.3%)

Other Asia
and Australia
(2.4%)

1990
Total imports: $3.3 billion

Canada
(2.8%)

Other
(21.3%)

EC
(45.9%)

Japan
(24.2%)

Other Asia
and Australia
(5.8%)

Note: 1980 figures exclude diagnostic products.

Figure 27. Major suppliers of United States medical products imports, 1980 and 1990.

Source: U.S. Department of Commerce. Reprinted from Health Industry Manufacturers Association, *Competitiveness of the U.S. Health Care Technology Industry* (1991), 15.

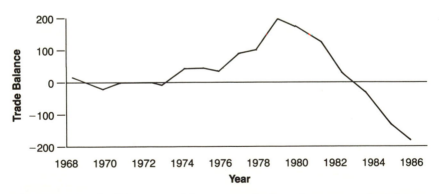

Figure 28. United States and Japan medical equipment trade balance (based on SIC categories).

Source: Susan Bartlett Foote and Will Mitchell, "Selling American Medical Equipment in Japan," *California Management Review* 31:4 (Summer 1989), 147.

Table 10. American and Japanese Medical Equipment
Consumption and Trade

| | U.S. medical equipment domestic purchases ($ billion) | U.S. global medical equipment trade balance | U.S. medical equipment trade with Japan ($ million) | | | Y/$ (real) | Japan medical equipment domestic purchases ($ billion) |
			Exports	Imports	Balance		
	(a)	(b)	(c)	(d)	(e)	(f)	(g)
1986	18.4	−0.01	355	526	−171	204	4.8
1985	17.1	0.2	279	396	−117	261	3.2
1984	16.1	0.4	260	282	−22	258	—
1983	14.6	0.7	243	217	26	254	—
1982	14.1	1.1	231	149	83	249	—
1981	12.2	1.3	258	110	147	212	2.8
1980	11.5	1.3	279	131	149	197	3.2
1979	11.8	1.2	314	130	185	197	—
1978	12.2	1.0	228	133	94	181	1.1
1977	11.5	0.8	193	110	83	205	1.1
1976	10.0	0.7	146	124	22	215	—
1975	9.5	0.7	128	95	34	206	—
1974	10.0	0.7	126	92	34	179	—
1973	9.3	0.5	92	97	−5	199	—
1972	7.9	0.4	59	62	−3	267	—
1971	7.0	0.4	41	43	−2	287	1.0
1970	6.4	0.4	37	46	−9	284	0.9
1969	6.5	0.4	31	35	−3	283	0.7
1968	6.0	0.4	27	20	6	278	—

Sources:

(a–b) Bureau of the Census, 1956–1986, 1967–1986

(c–e) Country market series

(f) Japan Statistics Annual, 1987

(g) Export Markets Digest, 1973; ITA, 1979; Pacific Projects, 1983, 1987

Reprinted from Foote and Mitchell, "Selling American Medical Equipment in Japan," *California Management Review* 31:4 (1989): 148.

Derivation:

(a) Domestic Manufactures plus imports minus exports (SIC 3693, 3841, 3842, 3843, 3851).

(notes continue on next page)

SELLING AMERICAN MEDICAL EQUIPMENT IN JAPAN

Some have argued that both trade barriers and exchange rates explain our declining balance of trade with Japan, but these are not the complete or even the primary explanations underlying medical equipment trade patterns between the two countries. The data indicate that sales of American equipment have been increasing in Japan. Japan imports at least as great a proportion of its medical equipment as does the United States (about 20 percent, compared to 15 percent in the United States). Despite adverse exchange rates, the American share of medical equipment imports to Japan grew from 30 percent in the early 1970s to over 60 percent in the mid-1980s.[3] The deficit has occurred because American purchases of Japanese manufactured goods have risen faster than American sales in Japan.

Obviously American firms need to preserve their competitive positions in their own marketplace, the largest in the world. However, American companies can also improve device sales in the Japanese market. The following discussion describes the key government policies in the Japanese medical market and then briefly analyzes why certain American products and firms have been successful in the Japanese market.

Safety Regulation as a Nontariff Barrier

Medical devices are subject to extensive government safety regulations in Japan. These regulations may have explicit or implicit effects on foreign producers.[4]

(notes from table 10 continued)

(b) Exports minus imports.

(c, d) Export and import equivalents of SIC categories in (a).

(e) (c) minus (d).

(f) Nominal yen/dollar times the ratio of the U.S. medical price index (1972–1986: OTA index for SIC 3693; 1968–1971: Producer Price Index) to the Japanese wholesale price index.

(g) Japanese medical equipment purchases net of trade. Converted at nominal exchange rates and deflated by the U.S. medical price index. Estimates not available some years.

All figures deflated by the U.S. medical price index as defined in (f), except as noted in (f).

There are no overt tariff barriers to the import of medical equipment into Japan. Ever since the Japanese government suspended the "Buy Japanese" program in the early 1970s, the most significant barrier to entry for medical equipment has been safety regulation. It has been argued that the Japanese Ministry of Health and Welfare (MHW) imposes nontariff trade barriers that discriminate against foreign producers in a protectionist manner.[5] While there is no evidence of explicit discrimination against foreigners, there has been concern about implicit barriers.

In 1961, Japan enacted the Pharmaceutical Affairs Law to control the marketing of medical devices and pharmaceutical products. To bring a product to market, all domestic and foreign producers must obtain either manufacturing or import approvals (*shonin*) of the product itself. The MHW issues *shonin* after consultation with the Central Pharmaceutical Affairs Council, which reviews the scientific data on safety and efficacy submitted by the applicant.

In addition to *shonin*, every producer must obtain a license to manufacture or import (*kyoka*) by presenting documentation that appropriate safety and manufacturing standards have been met. After the *shonin* and the *kyoka* have been obtained, the next step is to receive a price listing. The MHW sets prices for drugs and procedures involving medical equipment based on rules established by the Social Insurance Medical Affairs Council (Chuikyo).[6]

Until the late 1970s, Japanese medical equipment purchases were low. Many American firms had little interest in the Japanese market. As Japanese consumption of medical equipment increased in the 1980s, however, American exporters began to look seriously at the Japanese marketplace. In the process, they expressed frustration with the regulatory system. The two governments held trade meetings periodically from 1982 to 1985.[7] On 2 January 1985, President Reagan and Prime Minister Nakasone specifically identified pharmaceutical and medical equipment trade as one of four important sectors in the market-oriented, sector-selective (MOSS) talks that followed.

In January 1986, the U.S. and Japan MOSS negotiating teams issued a final report.[8] It addressed many issues related to uncertainties and delays in the regulatory process and the limited opportunities for producers to communicate with regulatory authorities. Even the Japanese industry supported proposals to streamline the regulatory bureaucracy. According to Koichi Ichikawa, President of the Japan Medical Equipment Manufacturers Association, "[T]he [Japanese] industry has nothing against the U.S. demands which are, for the most part, legitimate concerns regarding the approval-obtaining procedure. Considering that the procedural problem is shared by domestic manufacturers and importers, the industry recommends that the U.S. demands be accepted."[9]

Other issues raised in the MOSS negotiations were primarily of concern to foreign producers. The most important was the acceptance of foreign clinical test data as evidence of safety and effectiveness. Some American companies argued that the requirement that all clinical tests be done in Japan on resident Japanese citizens was designed to discriminate against foreign companies, requiring duplication of clinical testing and leading to delay in market entry.[10] The Japanese, however, believe strongly in their unique racial makeup. The government argued that these racial differences require validation of safety on Japanese people before marketing. Japanese negotiators in the 1983 talks refused to accept the arguments that foreign data provide sufficient safety information. In 1986, however, they made significant compromises. Under the MOSS agreement, except where there are demonstrable immunological and ethnic differences, foreign clinical data will be accepted for all examination and testing requirements but not for implantable devices, such as heart valves and pacemakers, or those products affecting organic adaptability.[11]

American firms also objected to restrictions on transfers of *shonin* from one business entity to another. American companies are considerably less stable than Japanese firms,[12] often changing ownership. Consequently, they expect flexibility in business arrangements, such as shifts in licensee or in place of operation or manufacture. The rules for transfer of *shonin* were quite rigid; any change in name or ownership required producers to obtain new approvals and prices with requisite delays and costs. The Japanese agreed to consider changes in these procedures.

Americans expressed guarded optimism that the MOSS negotiations would improve the situation for their firms.

Understanding the Medical Marketplace

A fundamental understanding of the health care system has been essential to successful penetration of the Japanese medical equipment marketplace. Japan has a combination of a public commitment to health and a fragmented private sector delivery system. Article 25 of Japan's constitution declares that promotion and improvement of public health, together with social security and social welfare, are the responsibilities of the nation.[13]

The Japanese medical system provides health coverage for virtually all of the population. The private sector delivers the services and is reimbursed by the government. In essence, payment is centralized, but delivery is fragmented. Thousands of autonomous hospitals and other medical institutions purchase equipment and supplies. In 1984 there were 181,000 doctors. By law, the head of a hospital must be a doctor; 76,000 physicians owned their own hospitals or clinics. Solo practice is the norm; hospital chains are rare. Relationships between hospitals are not close, and joint purchase of equipment is not common.[14]

Direct government control of purchasing decisions would be difficult or impossible in this system, but it can influence purchase and use decisions through the reimbursement system. The MHW has supplied generous resources to pay for technology, whether domestic or imported. For example, Japan, with half the population of the United States, has about the same number of CT scanners.[15]

There are restrictions on purchases. The MHW sets prices for all drugs and diagnostic procedures. In a system dominated by private practitioners, the incentives to provide these products are related to their profitability. The government sets the reimbursement price. Physician and laboratory profits are then determined by the difference between the government's rate and the price paid to purchase the drug or the device or to deliver the service, such as a diagnosis, using the device. By the late 1980s, price issues were highly controversial because the government began to contain costs by reducing reimbursement rates.[16]

MHW cost-control policies have restricted the ability of American and European firms to sell equipment to Japanese purchasers. However, the restriction has not occurred by direct fiat or even by an unstated preference in favor of Japanese manufacturers. Instead, the foreign manufacturers have usually charged more than Japanese companies for medical equipment and are not price competitive. The barrier is primarily the result of a foreign firm's inability or unwillingness to meet prices rather than an intended consequence of Japanese public medical care payment policy.

American Success in Japan

In addition to the Japanese government policies that present barriers to foreign firms, there are significant cultural differences in approaches to health and illness and in expectations about medical equipment. Language barriers can also be a problem.[17] In order to succeed in this fragmented but quality- and price-conscious market, foreign producers need innovative, cost-competitive products with efficient distribution systems. Japanese physicians respect innovation and often associate that attribute with American goods.[18] They have been willing to seek out foreign suppliers of innovative products even when the manufacturer's distribution system was weak.

Innovative American companies, such as SmithKline Beecham and Abbott Laboratories (through Dainabott, a joint venture with Dainippon Pharmaceuticals), have established strong leadership positions in clinical chemistry products (for example, blood analyzers, immunochemistry, and reagents).

American firms have an important edge in implant technology. Medtronic dominates the implanted pacemaker technology in Japan, with Cardiac Pacemakers a strong force also. Indeed, in pacemaker technology, several major Japanese firms, notably Toshiba, NEC, and Silver Seiko, tried to enter the field but have abandoned it. Knowledgeable observers speculate that these companies retreated because they lagged in technological and clinical know-how.[19] Market success, therefore, requires both a product that is mechanically reliable and a staff that understands its use.

Many of the new medical technologies that have diffused through the Japanese medical system have been simpler or cheaper than the best-selling versions in the United States. CT scanners, for example, were introduced into Japan in 1976, about three years after they were first sold in the United States, and are now in almost all hospitals. Most of the scanners, however, are head units, rather than the more expensive whole-body machines common in the United States. Magnetic resonance imagers, too, have diffused through the Japanese medical system. Most have been low-powered units selling for about $500,000 rather than the $2 million helium-cooled superconducting units that have sold well to American institutions. Japanese domestic firms may succeed because of lower production and capital costs.[20]

In addition to the product attributes described above, American firms must master marketing in the fragmented Japanese health care system. Sellers must possess sophisticated and well-developed distribution systems. Language barriers and cultural norms require a Japanese sales force. In turn, sales personnel need to develop stable, long-term relationships with the thousands of physicians who make the purchase decisions. Most foreign companies have been only partly successful in meeting these institutional demands. Direct investment in Japan is expensive and requires a long-term marketing commitment. Japanese purchasers, as well as potential employees, are skeptical of American firms because of the frequent mergers, acquisitions, and corporate reorganizations that characterized American industry in the 1980s.[21]

Some Japanese regulatory procedures continue to frustrate foreigners and have implicitly discriminatory effects. Government payment policies favor low-cost devices, often produced domestically. There is no substitute for familiarity with the language and the nuances of culture and tradition.

However, the barriers are not insurmountable. Sales of U.S. medical equipment in Japan have been increasing as the Japanese market has grown, from $128 million in 1975 to $355 million in 1986.[22] New medical equipment can ameliorate social ills and transcend ethnocentric trade concerns. Thus, while the Japanese regulatory system and the medical marketplace must be reckoned with, it does not create an impenetrable barrier to foreign medical devices.

THE EUROPEAN ECONOMIC COMMUNITY: UNCERTAINTIES FOR AMERICAN PRODUCERS

European Community Structure and Goals

Western Europe represents a substantial share of the global marketplace for American device producers. The twelve nations that comprise the European Economic Community (EC) include a population of over 320 million, most of whom are accustomed to fairly high-quality and highly technical medical care.[23] Collectively, the EC nations consume 16.4 percent of the world's medical equipment, ranking second in consumption, and purchase 39 percent of U.S. exports. The EC is also an important global competitor, producing 15.8 percent of all medical equipment.[24]

Many changes in this region were on the horizon in 1990. Indeed, the goal of the EC is unification by 1992. Unification includes the establishment of a common market with no barriers to trade for goods, services, and capital, including the free circulation of labor, the abolition of customs between member states, and the harmonization of regulatory policies among the states.[25] In pursuit of unification, all industrial product tariffs were abolished in 1977. Many nontariff trade barriers remained, such as conflicting national product regulations. During the 1970s, domestic economic problems in member states and increased competition in world markets reduced political momentum to achieve a unified European market. A new initiative began in 1985 with a detailed program of action that set 1992 as the deadline for a unified internal European market. Indeed, 1992 has become a rallying point for producers concerned about the future of the European marketplace.

The European Community is governed by a quadripartite institutional system consisting of the European Commission with executive powers, the European Council with legislative authority, the European Parliament (also called the Assembly), and the European Court of Justice. Policy-making functions are shared principally by the Commission and the Council, with the Assembly relegated almost entirely to an advisory role.[26]

Legislation emanating from these various institutions includes regulations, directives, and court decisions as well as advisory opinions and recommendations. Directives are the most relevant source of law for medical device producers and are formulated within the Commission and adopted by the Council. A directive is binding as to the result it prescribes, but it leaves national authorities the choice of how to achieve the required result. The private sector has some influence on the formulation of EC directives. Interested parties, such as manufacturers' associations, trade associations, and scientific groups, can assert the need for harmonized European legislation.

During the late 1970s and early 1980s, political differences between member states resulted in lengthy delays in the progress of integration. Reforms were passed to facilitate harmonizing legislation. One major change was that directives became mandatory. The council originally had adopted a concept of "optional directives," which permitted producers to choose freely between national standards and community standards if they had been developed. Another change permitted directives to set more general "essential safety requirements" instead of detailed technical specifications of production. Thus, individual countries could implement "technical standards," also referred to as "harmonized standards," to supplement mandated safety requirements as long as state standards conformed to the more general requirements.[27]

The Commission's "white paper," published in June 1985, contained three hundred legislative proposals to achieve economic integration. The white paper set out the general objectives, strategy, and philosophy for creation of the unified market.[28] It declared that there must be mutual recognition of product marketing and manufacturing standards among the states and that legislation harmonizing divergent standards must be enacted to ensure mutual recognition.[29]

To comply with the white paper, thousands of laws and regulations governing the production and the sale of goods and services had to be either abolished or unified and differences in technical standards and regulations had to be harmonized. In order to establish uniformity for technical standards, two European standardizing committees were established to elaborate technical standards for the operation and evaluation of testing laboratories and certification bodies. If they elaborate a specific technical standard, that standard must replace the relevant national standards. These committees—CEN (European Committee for Standardization) and CENELEC (European Committee for Electrotechnical Standardization)—have elaborated several specific standards, but many more will be required before harmonization is complete.

Harmonizing Medical Device Policies

The European Commission identified medical products as one of the sectors requiring action to complete the internal market by 1992. As in other industries, however, the creation of a common technical framework for medical devices has been difficult. As of 1990, four directives concerning medical devices had been proposed and were at various stages of the legislative process. The proposed directives would harmonize major differences between member nations regarding technical design specifications for medical devices and the administrative procedures for examinations, tests, and inspections and authorization required for their marketing and use.

Each directive addresses different sectors of the device industry. Four trade groups, corresponding to the types of devices in each category, have participated in drafting the proposed laws. The categories, types of devices included, and participating organizations follow.

1. Active implantable electromedical devices directive: devices surgically implanted into the human body for long-term purposes that require an electric power source, primarily pacemakers; International Association of Medical Prosthesis Manufacturers (IAPM).

2. Active, nonimplantable medical devices directive: devices that require a power source, for example, X-ray equipment

and diagnostic scanners; the Coordination Committee of the Radiological and Electromedical Industries (COCIR).

3. Nonactive medical devices directive: devices implantable or not, that do not need any power source, for example, heart valves and catheters; the European Confederation of Medical Suppliers Association (EUCOMED).

4. In vitro diagnostics directive: a combination of chemical products and devices that are used for analysis or diagnosis, such as home pregnancy tests and laboratory test equipment; the European Diagnostic Manufacturers Association.

In May 1990, the European Parliament approved the active implantable electromedical devices directive, which was sent to the European Council for a final vote. The nonactive medical devices directive is currently before the European Commission, where the main issue is product classification. The two other designated categories had directives in the early draft stages in 1990.

The directive for active implantable electromedical equipment provides some indication of the contours of medical device regulation. Member nations are directed to comply with the essential safety requirements that are quite broadly stated. In general, patients are to be "adequately protected" from risks related to sterilization, design, manufacturing, and other processes.[30] They will be protected through the development of harmonized standards, or relevant national standards should no harmonized standards exist, that are consistent with these broadly stated community goals. Manufacturers that comply can affix the EC (European Community) mark to their products, enabling devices to circulate anywhere in the internal market of 1992. Determination on compliance is left to national inspection bodies, which are required by the directive to be independent, expert assessment entities. Many details about these "notified bodies" are left to the individual nations.

The drafts of other directives seem substantially similar in form. The goals are identical; the differences relate to the variety of devices covered. For example, the draft on nonactive devices further divides the products by risk levels, in a manner reminiscent of the FDA's three-tiered classification system.

It is clear that the EC is struggling to develop a coherent, flexible, yet protective, medical device environment. However, a number of important questions are raised by these draft directives, some of which are discussed below.

"Safety" Is a Value Judgment

As we saw in chapter 4, the design of a regulatory structure for medical devices presented a difficult challenge for the United States. The European Community's efforts to harmonize regulations present an even greater challenge. In addition to accommodating the diversity of the devices themselves, the EC must harmonize the regulations among all member nations.

Many individual European countries have established safety regulations relating to drugs and medical devices. To a large extent, safety regulations reflect the values of a nation; how much it is willing to pay for a certain level of safety. As we have seen in our discussion of U.S. medical device regulation, there is no such thing as absolute safety—each nation's policies reflect an "acceptable" level of risk.[31] Some economists have noted that the "marketing of health care products, equipment, and services tends to closely follow national lines, due largely to national differences in attitudes toward drugs and traditions of medical practice."[32]

Indeed, this social value or cultural aspect of health-related products may explain why the EC's efforts to harmonize pharmaceutical regulations had met with little success as late as 1988.[33] While drugs and devices may not be the only products with safety values embedded in government policy—automobiles and other vehicles may also reflect different concepts of safety—the value issues cannot be ignored. Indeed, it is precisely these value issues that led the individual nations to impose different comprehensive pre- and postmarketing product requirements and that now make efforts to harmonize more challenging. Once the actual harmonization begins in earnest, how the general "essential safety requirements" will "adequately protect" patients may become considerably more controversial among member nations.

Standards and American Producers

The American experience would also suggest that a focus on standards might stultify innovation within the EC. Recall that although the FDA can require standards for all Class II devices, after thirteen years no detailed standards have been drafted. This dearth of regulatory standards is, in part, due to the cumbersome nature of the law's standard development process. However, there is no great push to develop standards because they reflect the state of the art only at the time they are written and are soon rendered obsolete in a dynamic industry.

American industry has tended to rely on voluntary, independent standard-setting organizations, such as the American National Standards Institute (ANSI) and the Association for the Advancement of Medical Instrumentation (AAMI), among others.[34] American firms have recognized that they must cooperate with the U.S. government to participate in the international standard-setting process. This voluntary, pluralistic approach is out of synchrony with the harmonized European system, which is leaning toward the imposition of technical standards as its primary regulatory mechanism.[35] If the EC adopts standards that are substantially different from those in the United States, producers could face extensive barriers to marketing their goods in Europe.

Will the Procedures Ensure Uniformity?

Achieving uniformity under the scheme as currently outlined in the directives will be very difficult. If EC standards take years to develop, devices will be subjected to national standards that comply with the vague "essential safety requirements" in the directives. Because member nations vary in their individual commitment to safety, uniformity may be an elusive goal.

Will These Directives Create Nontariff Trade Barriers?

Interested observers have many concerns about the consequences of European unity. Some fear that this large market will erect protectionist barriers that will disadvantage all non–

European Community competitors. European business and industry have pressured for the creation of a pan-European market, and they clearly hope to reap advantages from it. Some predict that as EC nations eliminate trade restrictions among themselves, they may transfer them to foreign market players.[36] Drawing on this large and protected internal market, European companies will drive out smaller, less competitive European companies and will seek to establish strength in the global marketplace. Requirements for local (EC) content, import quotas, and other tariff barriers could accomplish these protectionist aims.

There is also concern that internal efforts to harmonize regulations among the various nations will serve as nontariff trade barriers to outsiders. For example, product design standards could be constructed that are different from American or other international standards. The creation of an "EC" standard would benefit those whose primary market is internal. Observers fear that the considerable influence of European manufacturing interests in developing harmonized standards through the directive process will solidify the strength of insiders at the expense of outsiders. It seems fair to ask who is designing the internal requirements and standards. Some fear that the EC is farming out rule writing to standard-setting bodies that are overly influenced by European product designs rather than by U.S. or international designs.[37]

One early strategy of outsiders has been to participate in the development of harmonized product standards. Many large multinationals, including American companies such as General Electric, already have large European operations and have been active in the trade groups. However, smaller firms and latecomers may be disadvantaged if "fortress Europe" is realized. Some contradict the widespread view that established U.S. corporations would automatically have status equal to European companies.

The size of the U.S. market and the reputation of its medical device industry both operate in its favor. It would contradict any European global strategy if EC products did not comply with FDA requirements. The United States consumes more than half of all medical technology, a percentage that global strategies cannot ignore. Furthermore, the general European perception is that U.S. medical products are of high quality and reliability; FDA approval carries weight throughout the world.

There are additional reasons why Europe might not exclude foreign medical devices. Demand for medical products often transcends national, or in this case regional, lines. Inevitably, tensions will arise between the general economic goals of nations and the pressure for access to low-cost health care technology. Europeans are used to high-quality and comprehensive care. And the national governments are often the purchasers of health care products, particularly in some EC nations with comprehensive government-run health care systems, such as the British National Health Service. If EC regulations discriminate against foreign medical technology, then they would pose barriers to U.S. innovations that may be better and/or cheaper than European products. Once again a potential conflict emerges between an economic goal of supporting an industrial sector and the social and political goal of low-cost and effective health care services. Will member nations tolerate limits on choices in health care purchasing in the interests of economic growth?

THE CHINESE MEDICAL DEVICE MARKET

Chinese Health Policies

The Chinese medical marketplace illustrates how a government shapes both supply and demand for medical products. China also provides an opportunity to observe the interplay among the three major global competitors in the medical device market— the United States, Japan, and western Europe.

Chinese government policies determine the supply of imported medical technology and the size of the demand for it. Before 1978 the government strictly controlled imports and followed a policy of favoring domestic production. Hospitals and medical schools used little foreign medical equipment.[38]

Government policy changes in 1978 affected both supply and demand. On the supply side, a relaxation of import restrictions, a favorable climate for medical technology exhibits, and other forms of product promotion increased sales by foreign companies. On the demand side, more foreign exchange was made available for importation of western medical equipment. After the open-door policy of 1978, China acquired greater reserves of foreign exchange to implement the goal of improving available medical technology.

China's market structure makes it a complicated place to sell medical technology. The medical care system is substantially decentralized in terms of both high-level policy-making and delivery of services. A number of government agencies have authority over the diffusion of medical equipment, and disputes among them occur over tension between economic growth and health care services.

From the early 1950s until 1961, production and distribution of medical technology were overseen by several ministries, all of which were organized to promote economic growth (for example, the Ministry of Light Industry, the Ministry of Chemical Industry, and the Ministry of Mechanical Engineering). Between 1961 and 1978, the Ministry of Health oversaw medical technology. This ministry had a number of departments in charge of medical services, including administration, prevention, education, and financing. Unlike the other ministries, this one did not promote economic growth. The key medical schools and forty affiliated hospitals were directly under its supervision. The ministry controlled the procurement of medical equipment and provided medical technology information.

In 1979 the National Bureau of Medical and Pharmaceutical Management was established under the direct supervision of the State Economic Council. Within the bureau, the China Medical Instrument Corporation is in charge of policy, regulation, and guidelines on research, production, imports, and exports of medical instruments. Although they have substantially different missions, the Ministry of Health and the Bureau of Medical and Pharmaceutical Management must work together. The ministry, for example, must obtain a concurrence from the bureau for the importation of medical equipment to ensure that domestic products have not been overlooked. The Chinese government bureaucracy has tried to balance the goals of domestic economic growth with the growing demand for more sophisticated and technological western medical equipment.

Medical equipment sales depend on a very decentralized purchasing base. The government subsidizes hospitals in fixed amounts according to size. Hospitals rely on income generated from fees for services to make up the difference between government subsidies and expenditures. The local Price Bureau, an independent institution under the supervision of the State Economic Commission, sets the fees. Charges for new diagnostic tests with new equipment can be negotiated with the Price Bureau—a strong incentive to acquire new equipment and charge higher fees.

Each of the twenty-one provinces, five autonomous regions, and three metropolitan areas has its own health department that operates under guidelines from the Ministry of Health. These departments oversee the medical schools, the provincial hospitals, and the activities of local units but do not directly manage local hospitals and other health facilities.

Foreign Competition in China

Foreign competitors must operate within this labyrinthine marketplace. Overall consumption of medical and pharmaceutical equipment has risen dramatically in recent years, from $517 million in 1984 to $740 million in 1986, to nearly $1 billion in 1990.[39] This rise is attributed to the low level of medical technology at the beginning of 1984, the growing demand for medical care, the expansion of the economy, and the state policy to improve service at the provincial level. China's total budget for health care is expected to increase from $2.03 billion in 1987 to $2.49 billion in 1990. There has been a dramatic increase in imports, which grew at an 18 percent average annual rate between 1984 and 1986 and which account for approximately 57 percent of annual consumption. The area of largest growth appears to be in electromedical, radiological, and clinical lab equipment. The total import market is expected to be $530 million by 1990.

Who will get the largest share of this important market? In 1988, Japan had a market share of 33 percent, the United States had 24 percent, and West Germany had 9 percent. Equipment cost appears to be a major consideration. Japanese CT scanners are considerably cheaper than those of U.S. and German competitors and tend to dominate the market. Other important product attributes include the availability of training, service, and replacement parts. Some users indicated that more Japanese medical instruments have been adopted by Chinese medical institutions because the Japanese companies offer superior service.[40]

Chinese government policy plays an important role in shaping the market for medical device technology. Foreign competitors must confront domestic protectionist policies that have economic, rather than social, motivations. It is difficult to do business in this decentralized marketplace. Both domestic and foreign competition are strong in many market segments. Companies that understand the economic and social needs of the Chinese will succeed in this rapidly growing market.

American medical device producers once dominated the world market, and they cannot afford to be complacent about the future. Powerful competitors challenge innovative American firms at home and abroad. Major political, social, and economic changes threaten America's leadership in foreign markets. Successful exporters must understand complex governmental health and regulatory policies as well as the intricacies of tariffs and trade regulations. The world market contains as many uncertainties as the domestic market, and trends of the 1980s show losses for American producers abroad.

PART THREE
THE PROGNOSIS

Not everything that is new in health technology
is good; not all that is good is needed.

Stephan Tanneberger
"When Must a New Approach to
Treatment Be Introduced?"

9

MANAGING THE
MEDICAL ARMS RACE

In order to control the medical arms race, the policies that promote the flow of desirable innovations must be balanced with appropriate incentives that inhibit the production of unsafe technologies and the misuse or overuse of devices in the marketplace. Chapters 3 through 8 established the chronology of policy initiation and growth, outlining the evolution of public institutions and their interactions with the private sector. This chapter evaluates the consequences of policy proliferation. Recalling our analogy to polypharmacy, the discussion completes the brown-bag review.

This chapter is organized around the innovation continuum presented in chapter 1 (see figure 29). We can assume that desirable device innovations flow within the solid lines, all the way from the first idea to the patient's bedside. An appropriate policy mix would efficiently and expeditiously guide those products to the marketplace. Policies that restrict the flow, or allow them to spill over the banks, are unsuccessful.

The discussion in the chapter falls into three sections. The first provides an analysis of the present policy environment at both the discovery and the distribution stages, with illustrations of creative industry strategies that accommodate current policies. The second section discusses the pending and possible policy changes and their potential impact on the innovation stream. The third part addresses the interactions among the various public policies, which are inevitable consequences of policy proliferation. This part suggests mechanisms for elim-

POLICIES TO PROMOTE	R&D Funds ----------------->		Payment Policies ----------------------->
	Discovery		Distribution
POLICIES TO INHIBIT	<-------------------- Safety Regulation	<---------------------- Product Liability	<----------------------- Cost Controls Diffusion Controls

Figure 29. Policies affecting medical device innovation.

inating unnecessary duplication, reinforcing the effects of multiple policies, and encouraging coordination and cooperation among the relevant sources of policy, areas often overlooked by policymakers.

WHERE ARE WE NOW? DEVICE POLICY IN 1990

Promoting Discovery

As discussed in chapter 3, the 1950s ushered in an era of belief in the social benefits of scientific and technological innovation. Biomedical research was seen as the foundation for improvements in health care quality—permitting new understanding of disease and innovative treatment for illness. The creation of the National Institutes of Health represented a major federal commitment to support of biomedical R&D.

It is difficult to measure the overall impact of this federal research policy on medical devices. The relevance of basic scientific research to subsequently developed products is often hard to trace. As we saw in chapter 3, however, some research may be clearly directed to specific technological or device development. Throughout the last forty years, there has been tension between those who advocate NIH funding for basic science exclusively and those who favor targeted programs. In the last twenty years, there has been an increase in directed or targeted programs with contracts let to medical device firms. The directed research at the NIH tends to fall into disease categories (for example, cancer, AIDS, and cardiac disease), rather than device categories (for example, diagnostics or implants). For instance, NIH funding has supported innovation for treatment of renal diseases, which has led to artificial kidneys, dialyzers, and filtration systems, all of which are medical devices. However, not all supported research is disease-specific. Throughout the 1970s, NIH funded research on magnetic resonance imaging (MRI) systems, which can be used for diagnosis of many different medical conditions. The Small Business Innovation Research program also funds innovative private firms.[1] By 1982, however, industry was receiving only 6 percent of total NIH grants and contracts, and that sum included support for other activities in addition to medical device development.

The industry has not been dependent on federal funds for R&D support. The private sector has played an important role in supporting research and development. Particularly since the late 1970s, there has been a growing number of venture capitalists, specialists in providing financial capital to small firms, who have promoted innovators. However, venture capital is particularly sensitive to economic trends and tends to shy away from supporting projects where development costs are high and payoff is uncertain and longterm. Venture capital also considers the impact of future regulatory barriers—ease of entry encourages competition while premarket approval may be costly and time-consuming.[2]

Thus, NIH funds can serve as a bridge to support basic device research with the expectation that the private sector, through venture capital or other conventional fundraising efforts, will later oversee a project. In such situations, federal assistance can make or break a research project undertaken by a small firm. NIH refusal to fund can discourage research and development.[3]

Successful R&D Strategies: Novacor

NIH funding for the Artificial Heart Program illustrates the dramatic effects that government policy can have on particular firms. Novacor, a small innovative device company, owes its continued existence to NIH contracts. Dr. Peer Portnor, the founder of the company, is a physicist with experience in biomedical research. Like other entrepreneurial biomedical scientists, he gravitated to research areas where government funding was available, thus illustrating the impact of targeted programs on the focus of R&D.[4] The early work in his firm involved research in both the artificial heart, supported by the NIH, and gas analyzers, supported by NASA. Gradually, research came to focus primarily on the artificial heart, culminating in the 1978 formation of Novacor. Since that time the firm has received close to $20 million in NIH support. It has received some venture capital financing, but the long-term research agenda with limited commercial potential dampened the enthusiasm of early venture capitalists. Novacor was recently acquired by Baxter Travenol, but at least one-third of the firm's resources continue to come from the Artificial Heart Program.

Venture capital showed early interest in Novacor, but NIH support has been consistent over the longer term. Novacor's left ventricle assist device (LVAD), or the Novacor Heart Assist System, provides a bridge to transplant for suitable candidates. It keeps patients with failing hearts alive until a transplant can be performed. The firm is also working on a fully implantable permanent heart replacement for patients who cannot tolerate a transplant. The system is still in experimental clinical research at major university hospitals.[5]

The NIH is supporting a three-phase program for the fully implantable, electrically powered ventricle assist systems—device readiness, clinical evaluation, and patient follow-up. The first phase began in 1985. The AHP funded four groups of contractors, including Novacor, to run twelve LVAD systems for two years in a laboratory setting. At the second stage, the NIH planned to choose the two best preclinical performers for clinical trials. All three other firms experienced failures in the bench testing and dropped out of the trials. Two Novacor devices met the two-year performance testing requirement in December 1988. Consequently, Novacor was the only firm to receive a contract for the second clinical phase, with trials expected to begin in 1990 with fifty systems ready for implantation.[6]

For firms that are successful, the benefits of NIH targeted device development are clear. The AHP broke some of the traditional barriers to bioengineering that had developed at the NIH. But federal funds do not guarantee success. Many of the early innovators in the AHP did not survive despite federal support. Federal funds clearly can encourage certain avenues of research and can keep a research program alive when the private sector would have abandoned it.

In summary, there is widespread public acceptance of the federal government's efforts to support basic biomedical research. The direct federal policy promoting device discovery has been relatively modest. Device development is more likely to receive federal support if it can be used in the treatment of a disease that has been targeted by the NIH. The existence of NIH programs appears to spur and direct research in these areas as the story of Novacor indicates. The goal in many cases is to provide support for products not attractive to private capital because of long-term product development.

Inhibiting Discovery

The social motivation underlying federal regulation of medical devices was a desire for safer products. Following the controversies surrounding defective pacemakers and dangerous IUDs, it was clear that the public believed that the economic demands of the marketplace did not provide sufficient consideration of device safety. The prescription for this social ill was regulation, and the Medical Device Amendments of 1976 instituted an elaborate and comprehensive federal regulatory apparatus. Although the law covers all medical devices, its design intentionally focuses the highest level of scrutiny on a narrower group of high-risk devices.

Products requiring FDA premarket approval include devices for which sufficient data do not exist to ensure a reasonable degree of safety and efficacy. In practice, this requirement applies to less than 10 percent of all devices on the market. Devices subject to the requirement tend to be those that have serious consequences for patients if they fail. Examples include monitoring equipment and anesthesia delivery devices. Most implanted devices fall into the highest classification as well, including heart valves, pacemakers, ocular lenses, and prostheses. Another device category subject to premarket approval includes products that are significant breakthrough technologies about which little has been known before the innovation. One example is lithotripsy, the ultrasonic kidney stone crushing device; others include magnetic resonance imaging (MRI) and CT scanners.

All these devices represent the kind of important innovations that can improve the quality of care. The public desire for safety led to the creation of market barriers for all innovations. Producers must spend time and money to comply with FDA requirements. For example, experts estimate that the 3M Company budgeted in excess of $15 million for safety and efficacy trials associated with the cochlear implant. Total costs, of course, vary depending upon the device.

Complete data on the impact of federal regulation, particularly premarket approval requirements, have never been collected. Some research indicates that regulation may deter smaller firms from undertaking innovation or force them to abandon the field. The case study on cochlear implants discussed in chapter 7 is just one example of the difficulties of compliance with regulation. For the vast majority of producers, however, compliance involves reporting and recordkeeping requirements that may be annoying but that do not involve the significant costs and delays associated with premarket approval applications.

The second major policy is product liability, which is also a reflection of the value of safety. Product liability offers retrospective compensation for harms associated with a product, with an expectation that the consequences of a lawsuit will deter the future production of unsafe products. It is very difficult to predict the impact of product liability prospectively because court decisions vary from state to state and are subject to constant modification through common-law evolution and statutory amendments.

If one had to predict the likelihood of liability problems, the following categories of devices would be relevant. While regulation looks to the device itself, product liability predictions depend on additional environmental or situational factors. Products used by large numbers of patients have increased liability exposure; products used by certain classes of patients are more vulnerable than others. For example, young and otherwise healthy women injured by birth control devices invite sympathy from juries. Injuries to young children also generate large awards. Products used in high-risk procedures such as premature births, major surgery, or lifesaving situations are particularly vulnerable to litigation. The greater the risk to an otherwise healthy patient, the higher the likelihood that the technology will be implicated in an adverse court decision.

Regulation and product liability exposure target many of the same devices, but product liability has the additional consequence of proceeding case by case. Thus, one producer can face literally thousands of product liability suits with one product design failure. The case studies of pacemakers and the Dalkon Shield illustrate the devastating effects of mass lawsuits on the economic well-being of firms. However, even a small number of cases can be costly, and high expenses are incurred even when the producer prevails. Defending a successful case can run into tens of thousands or even hundreds of thousands of dollars. One punitive damage award can be several million dollars or more.

Creative Strategies: The IUD in the 1990s

The story of the IUD marketplace illustrates the effects of regulation and product liability on producers. As one might expect, producers will simply abandon the field if the environment is too threatening, as did several prominent IUD makers. Ortho Pharmaceutical withdrew its Lippes Loop in September 1985, and G. D. Searle halted U.S. sales of the Copper 7 IUD in January 1986. These two firms accounted for more than 95 percent of the IUD market at the time. Both cited business considerations, primarily lawsuits, not medical risks, as the reasons for withdrawal.[7] Since its first IUD went on the market in 1974, Searle had won thirteen of fifteen IUD related lawsuits that reached the trial stage. The two adverse judgments totaled about $300,000. The cost of fighting four suits was over $1.5 million in 1985 alone.[8]

Two smaller firms, however, recently developed creative responses to this less-than-optimal policy environment. Alza Corporation, a company that specializes in drug delivery systems, had offered an IUD that releases a birth control hormone. The IUD, known as Progestasert, entered the market in 1976. When Ortho and Searle left the field, Alza was the last firm selling IUDs in the U.S. market. It could have withdrawn as well. As a small company, it could ill afford major liability claims, and the Progestasert was not an especially important product in the firm's line. Alternatively, it could have aggressively marketed its product to seize market share.

Instead, Alza crafted a solution that would allow it to remain in the market while limiting its sales to women who would benefit from the product. The firm also consulted with women's health groups and legal advisers. The result is an unusually comprehensive program of physician and patient information. A patient counseling brochure requires potential patients to read and sign ten sections to indicate that they have discussed the material with the physicians and have read and understood the information. The physician or nurse is also required to sign a patient information form to indicate that counseling has taken place.

The firm has intentionally kept sales low—50,000 to 75,000 insertions a year. This number is significantly below the IUD market of over one million women in the mid-1970s. Responsible marketing has avoided sales to patients outside the recommended safety parameters, and detailed information helps to control potential liability suits brought on the basis of failure to warn of potential risks.[9]

A second firm followed in Alza's footsteps at the end of the 1980s. Concerned about declining research on contraception in the litigious environment of the United States, the Population Council, a nonprofit research group, developed an IUD that received FDA approval in 1984. The product was originally to be sold by Searle, but that arrangement fell through when Searle left the IUD market.[10] The Population Council then licensed the IUD technology to GynoPharma, a small start-up firm, in 1987. The firm submitted labeling and patient information to the FDA in 1988. ParaGard, the new product, is marketed with an extensive informed consent brochure modeled on Alza's document.

It is clear that regulation and product liability can have a powerful effect on the success or failure of medical devices. Products that are risky, even if they offer substantial benefits, must pass through significant FDA scrutiny. If they also have attributes that expose them to product liability (large patient base, high likelihood of harm to otherwise healthy individuals, for example), there can be additional potential barriers.

Balancing Promotion and Inhibition in Distribution

The present government policy toward distribution can promote or inhibit the flow of medical devices. As we saw in chapter 4, the advent of Medicare and Medicaid in the mid-1960s ushered in a period of expansion of health care services to large groups previously excluded from the system. The motivating social value behind these programs was a belief that there should be widespread *access* to the health care. The data indicate that medical technology sales soared following the advent of these government programs.

The policies of the 1970s and 1980s tried to contain or control costs associated with these federal and state programs. For some products, cost containment has not controlled market forces that encourage overdiffusion. When a policy works, however, cost containment protects the value of access by squeezing out unnecessary and wasteful expenditures incurred under the old cost-plus reimbursement system, expenditures that can lead to dangerous and unnecessary medical interventions. More cynical observers of HCFA's cost controls have argued that cost containment limits access and lowers the quality of care. The challenge has been to design a cost-efficient system that protects access without compromising quality. Results of the government's efforts to create a balance between the two have been mixed.

Thus, there was a new reality for medical device producers. There was the possibility of either a highly supportive or a very restrictive federal policy. When planning a new product introduction, the industry has had to learn how to manage given extreme market uncertainty. As politicians and bureaucrats tinker with reimbursement rules, device company managers have had to adapt rapidly to the idiosyncrasies of the regulated marketplace.

The impact on medical device technologies varies. Relevant factors include the costs of acquiring the technology, the costs of using the technology, the alternative treatments available, the location in which the device is used, and the effect of the device on outcomes (an increasingly important factor given the growing trend toward outcomes measures).

As indicated in figure 30, the most significant negative impact has been on cost-raising technologies. Technologies that increase quality while lowering costs (upper left quadrant) tend to survive, while those products that raise costs without increasing quality or reducing quality (lower right quadrant) would have a harder time in the present policy environment. Technologies that increase both quality and cost, however, face a very uncertain future. Ideally, if the incremental costs are worth the incremental benefits, the product should succeed. The challenge is to design policies that accomplish these goals. Our present policy environment does not always do so.

Both providers and producers have pointed out that assessing the costs of a technology before introduction and diffusion is problematic. Some have argued that if traditional cost-effectiveness analysis has been applied, the CT scan would never have been approved. Ultimately, CTs have been a cost-saving diagnostic technology that has dramatically increased the quality of medical care. At the very least, firms must now gather data to justify the costs of their products and would be well served by presenting information on the impact of their products on health outcomes as well. The need for research on the effectiveness of new technologies remains high. Policymakers have made only modest commitments to technology assessment.

Creative Strategies for Cost Control

Some firms have inaugurated creative strategies in this environment, striving to raise quality while minimizing cost. One ex-

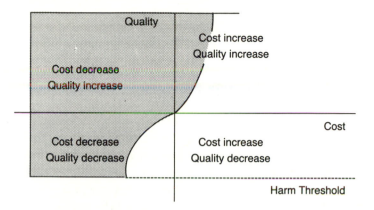

Figure 30. Impact of cost containment on medical technology. Shaded area represents positive effects.
Source: Nancy Cahill, esq.

ample is Acuson. Acuson designs, manufactures, and markets medical diagnostic ultrasound imaging equipment and has expanded sales throughout the 1980s. Its technology has several features that have helped it adapt to the cost-contained marketplace. The company's philosophy has been to develop products that are innovative, versatile, and capable of being upgraded or adapted to additional applications. For example, there are two major ultrasound imaging formats—sector and rectilinear. The former provides a wedge-shaped field of view, the latter a rectangular field. There are also three major ultrasound modes: imaging, Doppler (for analyzing blood flow), and M-mode (for cardiac analysis). Acuson's computed sonography system not only offers significantly better image quality but also provides films in both imaging formats and operates in all three modes. It can be upgraded primarily through software development without expensive investments in new hardware.

In 1985 and 1986, the firm added improvements without rendering its basic system obsolete or requiring customers to make major hardware changes. This flexibility allowed hospitals to acquire breakthrough technology efficiently. Acuson's system was identified as one of the products that "won big" in 1987.[11] Thus, it has managed to compete with a number of domestic firms, including major players such as General Electric and

Hewlett-Packard, as well such important producers in the international marketplace as Hitachi Instruments, Philips Ultrasound, Siemens Medical Labs, and Toshiba Medical Systems. Many of these competitors have significantly greater financial and other resources and compete in more market segments than Acuson.

As the discussion makes clear, some products have attributes that minimize the complications and the barriers of the policy environment. Low-risk, cost-reducing products find a hospitable marketplace. However, many of our most desirable innovations are expensive to develop, may bring high risks along with their benefits, and may raise costs. The failure of the cochlear implant illustrates the sensitivity of the device industry to public policy. If the market is perceived by the innovators as too hostile, then technologies will fall by the wayside. Indeed, there is evidence in some fields, such as contraception, anesthesia, and vaccines, that innovation has been adversely affected.

On the other hand, there is also evidence of overdiffusion in the medical marketplace, at least for some technologies. Overdiffusion leads to misuse and abuse of medical technology, adding unnecessary risks and additional costs to the health care system. This phenomenon occurs because of the attributes of the medical market and the limited ability of public policy to control market failures.

Demand for medical technology is enormous and often undisciplined by the market. Providers of care are attracted to new technologies because of economic incentives, professional pride, and peer pressure to be innovators and leaders in their field. These professionals, in turn, are pressured by equipment manufacturers who tout the virtues of their products and, on occasion, by patients who hear about new treatments in the media.

These groups often overlook costs. Patients with third-party coverage are insensitive to price, and providers expect reimbursement for services they perform. Moreover, traditional referral networks among specialists are often based on patterns of trust among professionals without reference to comparative costs of services provided. Sometimes, too, fear of medical malpractice drives providers to order additional tests and procedures.

Of course, excess demand can be constrained by limited supply. As we have seen, efforts to control supply through certificate-of-need programs in the states have been relatively unsuccessful. Supply can also be controlled by third-party payers. If the payers refuse to cover a new procedure or technology, that treatment will effectively not be available to patients. Medicare and Medicaid are large payers that have an impact on market supply. As we saw in chapter 7, Medicare coverage policy is decentralized and fragmented. Regional carriers are subject to pressures from patients and providers demanding access to new procedures and technologies. Under pressure, these payers tend to cover the desired procedure.

Once covered, third-party reimbursement rates become crucial. As we have seen in the case of cochlear implants, a disadvantageous pricing decision can destroy a technology. Conversely, expectation of high profits often encourages overuse and misuse, as the case studies of the pacemakers and intraocular lenses illustrate.

Public payers are hampered in their coverage and payment decisions by inadequate information. Assessment of the costs and benefits of new technology is problematic. The need for more information on the effectiveness and costs of new technologies is high; the federal government has been unwilling to invest sufficient resources for assessment.

And, once profitability of a procedure is established, greed often follows need. Acquisition of equipment or special skills associated with a new technology or procedure create economic pressures. There is increasing evidence of supply-induced demand, particularly where demand can be manipulated by physicians and hospitals anxious to turn a profit on new equipment. Examples of excess supply include the proliferation of CT and MRI equipment and the overcapacity of mammography screening devices. The aggregate data support a conclusion of overdiffusion, since the United States alone consumes about one-half of the world's supply of medical technology.

This vicious cycle of demand fueling supply, then supply inducing demand is what constitutes the medical arms race. Public payers, such as HCFA, can affect this process, although its market share is too small to exert a strong influence. Congress and HCFA have demonstrated neither a sufficient understanding of this process nor the political will to constrain providers and producers.

WHERE ARE WE GOING? CHANGING PRESCRIPTIONS THROUGH POLICY REFORM

Reformers obviously believe that there are some problems in the policy environment and seek to correct them. To understand motives for policy reform, we need to evaluate all the essential components of the problems, from the initial symptoms to the present cures. The *symptoms* are the social problems perceived when behavior in the private sector conflicts with shared social *values,* such as a desire for safe products or quality health care. Public *policies,* or prescriptions, are the government's way of imposing those values on the private sector. The manner in which the policies are crafted and implemented leads to *effects* on the device industry. These effects may be further influenced by the *interactions* of various policy prescriptions.

Treatment options depend upon an interest group's evaluation of each step of the inquiry. If reform is proposed, is it because the effects of the policy were unanticipated? If an effect is undesirable, is it because of a flawed policy design or a failure of implementation? Reform proposals often call into question the underlying values that first generated the policy.

This section will describe the various policy reform proposals under consideration in 1990. Several important themes emerge. First, there appears to be nearly unanimous acceptance of the federal government in all the areas under discussion; no viable interest group advocates that it abdicate its various roles. Thus, government participation in all aspects of device innovation is now legitimate. Second, there is little coordination among the described proposals. The effect of policy interactions, an important concern for polypharmacy, is generally overlooked in the present policy environment. Moreover, different interest groups dominate different policy reform arenas, so that greater inconsistencies in policy may well arise over time.

Policy Reform at NIH

The NIH is fully accepted as a legitimate supporter of biomedical research. However, there is controversy about how much funding to allot to the NIH and how to allocate money among the many competing areas of research.

NIH funding requires congressional authorization. In addition, the National Cancer Institute and the National Heart, Lung, and Blood Institute require specific periodic reauthorization. Budget debates at the NIH are constant and highly political. At any given time, the NIH is concerned simultaneously with spending its current budget, steering proposals through the executive and legislative branches, and developing a budget for the next funding cycle.[12] The battles over budget size can be bloody. For example, the Reagan administration consistently tried to cut back congressional proposals for NIH increases. When the NCI and the NHLBI came up for reauthorization in 1985, President Reagan twice vetoed reauthorization measures, only to see his second veto overridden by huge margins (380–32 in the House and 89–7 in the Senate).[13]

The medical device industry is generally supportive of large NIH budgets. During the 1989 Senate hearings on the NIH budget request, Frank Samuel, then president of HIMA, testified in support of the requested funding level of $8.2 billion. He acknowledged the debt of the industry to the NIH by listing innovative products that NIH funding supported. He specifically mentioned the Small Business Innovation Research Program (SBIR) as beneficial to the device industry.[14] The device industry favors programs targeted to firms but has not challenged the basic research performed at the NIH.

There is no compelling demand for major NIH reforms from any quarter: no general outcry for more money for medical device technology research or concern over the general types of research supported by the NIH. However, issues concerning American capacity for innovation have been voiced in relation to technology in general. It is possible, indeed likely, that innovation may be affected by cost containment in the public and private sectors, which will reduce corporate profits and R&D

expenditures. The recession of the early 1990s may also limit the ready availability of private venture capital funds, particularly if short-term profitability of new technology is limited. In order to enhance competitiveness and encourage innovation in such an environment, pressure may grow for greater government involvement.

This pressure could take several forms. First, there may be a push for more money for technology research within the existing NIH framework, such as more targeted funds for specific technologies not being aggressively developed in the private sector. Congress could create a new institute for medical technology development at the NIH that could coordinate and oversee the medical device research being performed there. While some oppose proliferation of institutes at the NIH and others see devices as simply part of the disease-oriented institute structure, more coherent technology research is needed at the federal level. This need, as we have seen, may deepen in an economic environment not conducive to innovation. How such an institute might interact with other federal institutions will be discussed later in this chapter.

Policy Reform at FDA

The value of *safety* underlies liability and regulation. The debate at the federal level about FDA regulatory reform has been dominated by members of Congress determined to tighten the regulatory rules applicable to devices and supported by proconsumer organizations such as Nader's Health Research Group. They assert that the FDA has failed to implement the 1976 law adequately and that the agency should administer a stronger dose to the industry. The 1990 Safe Medical Devices Act discussed below is the result of years of pressure to reform device regulation. In contrast, the trend in product liability reform is to provide greater protection for business interests generally and for drug and device firms specifically. Probusiness interests rarely assert that injured individuals do not deserve compensation; rather, they argue that the liability prescription has adverse side effects and needs major alteration. They look for procedural and substantive changes in the system that will reduce industry exposure to claims and the amount of awards available. On the other side, consumer groups and trial lawyers defend the present system. While no major liability reform has taken place in either the states or the federal government, limits on liability are often introduced. By the end of 1990, the reform environment looked inhospitable for device producers, with new regulation and no liability relief.

HR 3095, called the Safe Medical Devices Act, passed on 26 October 1990 and was signed into law by President Bush on November 17. Its original sponsors were Congressmen Henry A. Waxman and John D. Dingell, both powerful leaders in the field of product safety, health, and the environment.[15]

When the bill was first introduced, it was accompanied by strong language challenging the credibility of both the device industry and the regulatory zeal of the agency. Representative Dingell described "the sorry inability of the FDA to implement the 1976 medical device law as Congress intended. The result has been that the health of the American public has been jeopardized. Indeed people—young babies, the elderly, and men and women in the prime of life—have died because unsafe medical devices have been allowed on the market without scrutiny."[16] Representative Waxman echoed this perspective: "It must come as an unhappy surprise to many to hear that, in 1989, we have no assurance that the medical devices used in, on, and around our bodies are safe."[17]

Why is the device industry on the defensive in Congress? There are many possible explanations. First, there have been several serious allegations against some manufacturers for careless manufacture and design, including defective infant monitors.[18] However, none of the device problems has generated the kind of public concern that the generic drug industry scandals have in the same period.[19]

Furthermore, the device industry has not been very effective in counteracting congressional pressure, in part because of the fragmented nature of the industry—the diversity in firm size, in the focus on device products, and in the variations among the products themselves. This diversity often leads to a lack of a unified lobbying effort. Indeed, during the negotiations on the device legislation, some HIMA members broke away from the organization. Sources reported that three HIMA members derailed negotiations with Dingell's oversight subcommittee, and counsel for the subcommittee alleged that the association had failed to represent the interests of all of its members. The subcommittee threatened to exclude HIMA from subsequent discussions on proposed legislation. HIMA claimed that it was trying to ensure consensus. However, the organizational infirmities within the association were quite evident.[20]

The principal purpose of the new law was to strengthen the Medical Device Amendments of 1976.[21] The legislation contains many specific provisions, but all either increase FDA oversight and control of the device industry or streamline the detailed and often cumbersome provisions of the 1976 act. In the first category are provisions to increase the civil penalties that can be assessed against manufacturers for violations of the act, requirements for postmarket surveillance for permanent implants that pose serious risks or support human life, expanded reporting requirements, including the extension of mandatory reporting to "user facilities." These are defined to encompass hospitals, nursing homes, ambulatory surgical centers, and certain other outpatient facilities. The new law also makes it more difficult for a manufacturer to enter the market under "substantial equivalence" without the submission of safety and effectiveness data and codifies other current FDA practices.

The more cumbersome Class II requirements have been streamlined, with rigid performance standard requirements giving way to more flexible "special controls." Performance standards are made discretionary, not mandatory, and the process is more efficient. The 1990 law addresses many details of FDA regulatory authority. Much was delegated to the agency. Exactly how the agency will implement the new law, how it will allocate resources, and whether it will emphasize enforcement or efficiency depend on many factors. At best, the medical device industry is left with additional regulatory uncertainty.

Reform of Product Liability

The trend toward greater regulation is in stark contrast to the politics of product liability reform. As we saw in chapter 6, product liability rules derive from state court decisions and state legislative enactments. Product liability exposure can vary significantly among jurisdictions. However, the trend in virtually all the states is to limit the expansion of product liability that occurred in the 1970s. In addition, there are proposals to create a new federal product statute that would preempt state laws.

The press for reform in the 1990s derives from the perception of an insurance crisis that prevented producers from acquiring adequate and affordable coverage. The perceived crisis arose because of the massive expansion of liability standards, an explosive growth in the number of lawsuits, and increases in the size of jury awards in the 1970s.[22] In 1990, there was no consensus on the severity of either the liability or the insurance crisis.[23]

Despite the disputes about the real impact of liability, business and insurance interests have kept up a steady pressure to reform the system, particularly in the area of product liability. There have been notable successes in state legislatures. As of 1990, thirty-nine states had passed some form of liability reform,[24] including more procedural hurdles for plaintiffs, limits on punitive damages, and narrower definitions of the concept of defect. All are designed to provide more protection from liability for corporate defendants.

Reforms in some states related specifically to drugs and devices. The most directly relevant provision is known as the "government standards" defense. For example, New Jersey's tort reform statute provides that drugs, devices, food, and food additives that have received premarket approval or are licensed or regulated by the FDA shall not be subject to punitive damages unless the product manufacturer or producer knowingly withheld information or misrepresented the product during the approval process.[25] Another provision in the New Jersey law provides a presumption that any FDA warning is adequate, thus weighing the evidence in favor of a producer who has allegedly failed to adequately warn the user of the product's risks.[26]

Federal legislation to establish a uniform set of national rules for product liability legislation has been introduced in Congress every year for ten years. Two bills were pending in 1990. If passed, the legislation would preempt state law and require state courts to enforce the federal provisions instead.

Of course, the provisions of each particular piece of legislation vary. The Product Liability Reform Act (Senate bill 1400) serves as an example of federal efforts at product liability reform. Of particular relevance to the device industry is the government standards defense, similar to the New Jersey rule discussed above. Because of the experience of Dalkon Shield claimants, previous bills had included bars to government standards defense for contraceptive drugs and devices. Indeed, a bar to the defense had been proposed in, but was removed from, S. 1400. A number of bills are pending in 1991 to reform medical malpractice; at least one includes medical product reform as well.[27]

Because there is considerable uncertainty about the future of reform at the federal level, predictions about the next decade are risky. However, the interest groups that will fight this battle in the 1990s are clearly defined. The device industry is allied with a broad coalition of manufacturers and insurers, all of whom exert a substantial influence at both the state and the federal levels. Consumer groups and trial lawyers, who are particularly well-organized and vociferous opponents to reform, are arrayed on the opposite side. One tactic has been to challenge state product liability reform in the courts. For example, opponents of reform have challenged the constitutionality of state imposed caps on damage awards, with mixed results. Review of the constitutionality of punitive damages was pending before the U.S. Supreme Court in 1990.[28]

Device producers will benefit if the government standards defense is widely adopted in states or imposed on all states through federal legislation. The government standards defense provides a link between two very different institutions—the FDA and the courts—and recognizes the interaction between these two divergent sources of public policy. However, either institution can change its requirements without the other adjusting its rules. If the FDA alters its requirements for premarket approval, the justification for the government standards defense may weaken. As of 1990, however, device producers have more regulatory hurdles, including risks of substantial civil penalties for failure to comply, without any corresponding liability relief. Coordination among policies has not been considered and appears to have been overlooked.

The problem of policy proliferation is that there seems to be little formal or consistent coordination among the diverse sources. Whether one supports or opposes the new proposals is based on a value judgment—do they, or do they not, produce sufficient levels of safety, without undue impacts on cost, access, or innovation. The solution will be political, and it will turn upon the power of interest groups to influence Congress.

Policy Reform at Distribution

The value underlying government payment programs is access to health care services. Ideally, cost-containment policies do not threaten the value of access but only keep out waste and excess. The impact on technology producers is mixed: government payment supports use and government cost containment inhibits it. There is the possibility of either promotion or inhibition as government policies try to balance the goal of access within a cost-contained system.

As we have seen, federal and state payers have become the gatekeepers for many categories of devices. The categories most affected by government policy include products used primarily by elderly Medicare beneficiaries, expensive capital equipment used in hospitals, and devices that indisputably raise costs.[29] The larger the Medicare market share, the more dependent the producer is on decisions by HCFA. For producers with some Medicare market, HCFA's decision can influence, but not control, the other private third-party payers. If HCFA or its carriers refuse to cover a particular technology, the private payers may feel less compelled to do so for their policyholders. As we have seen in our case studies, some devices have been adversely affected by government reimbursement decisions. Of course, others such as pacemakers and IOLs have significantly benefited by government policies, although cost containment will probably affect all technologies to some degree.

The politics of reform affecting device distribution are significantly different. In contrast to the more comprehensive legislative proposals for regulatory and/or liability reform, it is unlikely that there will be a major overhaul of public payment programs.[30] It is also unlikely that any change would specifically benefit medical technology producers. The pressure to contain costs is simply too strong.

Device producers have been disadvantaged by cost containment. However, many powerful private and public interests want to see medical costs controlled and reduced. While insurers and producers are on the same side of the debate over product liability reform, insurers who pay the bills lobby heavily for cost containment. Hospitals and employers are also feeling the crunch.

The pharmaceutical industry remains a lukewarm ally because it has not yet been significantly affected by federal government programs.[31] The real allies of device firms in this context are consumers, who individually want access to all available alternatives, no matter how costly.[32] The medical device industry has not embraced consumer groups, no doubt because of suspicions stemming from their adversarial relationship in the product liability and the regulatory reform arenas. Alliances between the device industry and physicians vary, depending on whether the new device replaces doctors' services or otherwise affects a preferred practice pattern. In other words, the adversaries are very powerful, and the allies are only fair-weather friends. And unanimity among firms is difficult to achieve because the impact of payment policies varies depending on device characteristics.

Periodically, there are calls for reform within the DRG system. Suggestions include the creation of technology-specific DRGs and partial or temporary exemptions from DRGs for new technologies (reimbursement on the old cost-plus system for short periods of time, for example). Advocates, however, often admit that there is considerable risk that the cost-control mechanisms will be defeated by these types of exceptions.

For the most part, the political stance of device producers has been to manage within the system rather than to seek to overhaul it. Recall the efforts of Acuson to craft flexible locations and uses for their products. These efforts are case by case, as manufacturers try to persuade the HCFA to cover their products and place them in profitable DRGs. Recently, the strategy has been to generate information on the costs and the benefits of the new technology for government. The industry has given up opposition to data gathering through technology assessment. Instead, it has been willing, albeit reluctantly in some cases, to participate in technology assessment programs. In other words, the goal is to prove how beneficial (and cost effective) the new product is rather than to defeat cost containment. Manufacturers have been increasingly willing to take their case to the public, hoping that public pressure for desirable technologies can be exerted against government gatekeepers at the HCFA.

Given the realities of cost containment, producers of cost-increasing technologies will continue to face many inhibitory pressures on product adoption and diffusion. There is virtually no likelihood that comprehensive reform efforts could restore the price insensitive, technology consuming environment of the late 1960s and early 1970s. However, the present HCFA coverage and pricing policies are seriously flawed. We have seen many examples of both overdiffusion and underdiffusion because of HCFA decisions. HCFA needs more flexibility so that it can experiment with coverage alternatives, and it needs more information about the costs of new technologies. Coverage and payment reforms are necessary and should be forthcoming in the 1990s as Congress begins to focus on the medical arms race.

UNDERSTANDING INTERACTIONS

There is no reason to believe that multiple policy interventions per se are necessarily bad for the industry or those the industry serves. However, our brown-bag review considers possible adverse interactions among the various policies, and interactions could be improved at several points. Figure 31 identifies the areas of interaction discussed in this section.

One interaction occurs when two policies create overlapping, duplicate, or conflicting incentives (see *A* on figure 31). Both regulation and product liability are premised on the value of safety, yet their many differences—institutional, procedural, and methodological—lead to potential adverse reactions. Following a description of the interaction, a range of treatment options are presented.

Another form of interaction occurs when policies have similar goals but operate at different stages of innovation (see *B* on figure 31). That is, government regulation and government

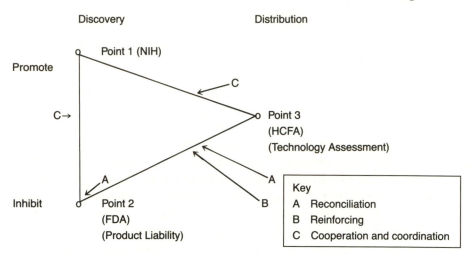

Figure 31. Policy interactions.

payment both may inhibit the flow of devices, but for different reasons. Reinforcing strategies can be developed to ensure that the policies do not operate at cross purposes but instead mutually support one another. Policies could be realigned to reinforce each other. The Pacemaker Registry, which is described below, is an example of reinforcing strategies, linking compliance with FDA regulation to favorable government payment and coverage decisions.

Finally, an interaction occurs when policies to promote devices confront policies to inhibit them (see *C* on figure 31). Examples include situations in which NIH promotion of innovation runs up against FDA requirements for safety and efficacy or in which NIH promotes devices for which HCFA may refuse to pay. Formal or informal mechanisms to ease the conflict or potential conflict at these points are possible. These efforts are characterized as coordination or cooperative strategies.

Reconciliation Strategies: Product Liability and Regulation

There is no fundamental reason why two or more prescriptions cannot serve the same goal. Controlling high cholesterol counts might require both dietary modification and a cholesterol lowering drug; treating coronary artery disease might require both medication and surgical intervention. Similarly, in the policy arena, it is possible to have more than one policy serving the same goal without conflict.

Product liability and regulation both support the underlying value of product safety. Yet the prescriptions to accomplish that goal are very different on many dimensions. First, and quite important, the two policies define the standards of safety differently. Regulators at the FDA are concerned with public health; its staff is composed of scientists, aided by advisory panels of independent experts. The agency evaluates products prospectively by reviewing laboratory and clinical data developed by the manufacturers. The agency can monitor the products after marketing, requiring reporting of adverse reactions, and if a product later proves unsafe, it can be removed from the market. In essence, the FDA's safety determination is scientific and primarily prospective. The validity of its decisions depends upon accurate information presented both before and after marketing.

The product liability system determines safety quite differently. The evaluation is retrospective, after the harm has occurred and the plaintiff has sued. The injured individual presents his or her claim to a jury of laypersons, not scientists, although scientific experts can testify on certain points. Many of the findings depend upon legal, not scientific, determinations. For example, the legal concept of causation of harm is quite different from the scientific concept of causation.[33] In most jurisdictions, compliance with FDA requirements for marketing is no defense against a legal determination of defect (that is, a product is unsafe).

Second, the two systems overlap. Regulation tries to deter the production of unsafe products through premarket and postmarket controls. The FDA has substantial powers to impose civil and criminal penalties. Liability law also protects society through its intended deterrence function. Arguably, producers are deterred from producing defective products through fear of subsequent product liability suits. However, liability law also compensates individuals for harms incurred from unsafe products and has the capacity to punish producers as well.

The existence of the two overlapping systems produces contradictory incentives for industry. The social function of regulation depends on information—gathering data before marketing and reporting problems once the product has been distributed. Without adequate and accurate information, the safety goals cannot be met. On the other hand, the threat of product liability suits intimidates producers. Even for manufacturers who are exonerated after a trial, the costs of defending a suit can be quite high. Thus, there are powerful incentives, even for responsible producers, to protect or to withhold information. And because compliance with FDA requirements is no defense to a product liability action, there are even fewer incentives to comply with the regulators.[34]

Finally, complying with regulation and defending against product liability actions (through insurance or costs of litigation and payments of awards) can be very expensive. As we noted in previous chapters, producing the required premarket approval data and complying with reporting and notification requirements can be very costly to a company. Of course, the decision to regulate concedes that the costs are worth it to achieve the desired level of safety. However, product liability is also expensive, and many of the costs associated with the system are procedural. Only a small percentage of the actual amount spent is transferred to the plaintiff if he or she prevails. Supporters of this system also maintain that the social costs of accidents should be covered by producers. The traditional justification is that producers can raise prices to cover the true social costs of their products.

In medical technology, however, policymakers cannot be cavalier about costs. Indeed, the costs of health care present a significant social issue in their own right. Medical devices are an integral part of the health care system. Costs associated with the public demand for safety must be evaluated against the equally pressing demand for widespread access to advanced medical technology and the undeniable cost pressures that all third-party payers face. The imposition of any unnecessary additional cost on a medical product is unacceptable. The imposition of too many barriers can deter innovation as well. This has already occurred in contraceptive and vaccine technology. Thus, we must be very confident that the systems support the fundamental value of safety and that they are worth the costs that they impose.[35]

Can safety be protected while streamlining the two systems? Can costs of these policies be reduced? Several alternatives are possible.

One response is to support the government standards defense in product liability actions. This defense presumes that the FDA definition of safety is adequate. FDA critics are likely to oppose the substitution of its definition for that of the courts on the grounds that the FDA has failed in its mission. The benefit of a government standards defense is that it allows the systems to remain generally intact and does not require a massive overhaul of long-standing institutions. The problem, of course, is that keeping the systems intact preserves their other problems, including the facts that costs remain high (cases must be defended) and that information disincentives continue to exist.

Another alternative is to support more extensive national product liability reform to ensure uniformity at the federal level.

A more drastic solution would be a formal merging of regulation and liability into a single regulatory/compensatory system. A detailed proposal integrating the safety goals of both institutions has been presented.[36] Such a plan is a variant of other compensation programs, such as state workers compensation plans that provide no-fault awards for work related injuries. Streamlining and controlling the impact of liability law on innovation characterizes the National Childhood Vaccine Program and forms the basis of recommendations to protect AIDS vaccine development from liability law that would deter innovation.[37]

Supporters of compensation programs generally assert that there are serious flaws in the judicial system that hurt both plaintiffs and defendants. They go beyond a critique of the costs of the system, alleging that arbitrary factors such as geography, quality of lawyers, and wealth of defendants result in similarly situated plaintiffs receiving very different awards.[38] They find only a capricious relationship between the amounts that plaintiffs recover and the seriousness of their injuries. In addition, there are long delays and risks of no recovery for injured people. Liability is expensive, and less than half of the premiums paid for liability insurance go to compensation.[39]

One major goal of a unified regulatory/compensatory system would be elimination of conflicting incentives for product producers. The manufacturer would receive benefits for compliance with the FDA so that the flow of information on adverse reactions would be unhindered, providing greater safety for the consumer. Compensation could be made more uniform, predictable, and expeditious. Limits on awards would reduce the costs to producers overall and would encourage certainty and predictability without sacrificing the compensatory function of the law. Procedural efficiencies would reduce costs, allowing for lower product prices and reducing the risk of deterring innovation.

It would be naive to assume that such a system would be easy to construct or that there would be no opposition from powerful political forces. But if we recognize the inefficiencies and inequities of policy proliferation, we must remain receptive to alternative solutions.

Reinforcing Strategies: Regulation and Payment

There are situations in which two government policies inhibit technology for different purposes. Can these programs reinforce their diverse goals?

Congress recently enacted the Pacemaker Registry, which is an excellent example of the use of reinforcing strategies. The Pacemaker Reimbursement Review and Reform was an amendment to the Deficit Reduction Act of 1984.[40] The goal was to obtain more information on pacemaker performance, and the law requires health care providers, as a condition of Medicare payment, to submit pacemaker information to an FDA registry. It permits the FDA to require that providers return explanted devices (devices removed from a patient after implantation) to the manufacturer and that manufacturers test returned devices and share the test results with providers.

The purpose of the registry is to aid the federal payment program in determining when Medicare should pay for pacemaker implantation or explantation, assessing the performance of pacemakers and pacemaker leads, determining when manufacturers should inspect their pacemakers or leads, and performing studies on these devices. The data collected must include the following: manufacturer, model, and serial number of the pacemaker; the date and location of the implantation or removal; any express or implied warranties for the pacemaker or leads; the patient who received the device; the physician who implanted or removed the device; and the hospital or other provider who is billing Medicare for the procedure. Reporting information to the registry will be required only if Medicare is requested to pay for the pacemaker, and the bill applies only to devices implanted or removed after the effective date of the implementing regulations. The law authorizes the FDA's Center for Devices and Radiological Health (CDRH) to require that FDA personnel be present while the manufacturer tests Medicare covered devices that may have failed.

The idea for this joint program developed as problems with pacemaker performance grew. The FDA funded a pacemaker registry at University of Southern California Medical Center from 1974 to 1981. The purpose was to gather experience data on pacemakers. Five medical centers participated, and the program included data on two hundred models of pulse generators produced by sixteen manufacturers. The original contract applied only to pacemaker pulse generators, but it was expanded in 1979 to include information about pacemaker leads. The data gathered by centers funded by the FDA supported the 1982 congressional investigations of fraud and abuse in the pacemaker industry.

The Center for Devices and Radiological Health set up a task force to determine how to proceed with the registry and to coordinate its efforts with HCFA. On 6 May 1986, HCFA and FDA proposed regulations for the registry.[41] Data in the registry could cover 170,000 to 200,000 devices each year. The FDA deferred development of regulations for certain discretionary sections of the act until the agency had some experience with the actual functioning of the registry.

In 1987, HCFA and FDA published a final rule implementing the national registry.[42] Under the rule, physicians and providers of services must supply specified information for the pacemaker registry each time they implant, remove, or replace a pacemaker or a pacemaker lead in a Medicare patient. If the information is not submitted, the HCFA can deny payment. The FDA gets the data to monitor the long-term clinical performance of pacemakers and leads. The registry is used together with the more general medical device reporting (MDR) regulation to track failures or defects in certain models and to notify HCFA so that they may stop Medicare payments for those models.

There is no doubt that pacemakers provide important benefits to certain patients. Medicare pays for about 85,000–100,000 pacemaker implants and replacements every year, which account for a large percentage of Medicare costs. Pacemakers have also been linked to serious medical complications as well as to fraud and abuse in the payment system. The HCFA/FDA plan allows the efforts of each agency to reinforce the other's: linking payment to safety information both improves regulation and reduces fraud. Similar linkages ought to be considered for other high-risk, expensive, but highly beneficial, medical technologies.

Cooperation and Coordination: Promotion and Payment

Another policy interaction focuses on the relationship between programs that promote and programs that inhibit device flow. The NIH is the primary agency charged with promoting medical device discovery, and it has interacted with other federal agencies whose goals include inhibiting medical devices for a variety of reasons.

The NIH can interact with the FDA. If the NIH funded only investigator-initiated projects, there would be little opportunity for contact with the regulatory agency, which reviews the product only in its later stages of development. However, for some targeted programs, the NIH has become involved in designing clinical trials and supervising product testing activities. In these cases, the researcher may discover that the FDA has a strong interest in the design and progress of the trials. Occasionally turf battles erupt if the FDA disapproves of a trial design that has been developed in conjunction with the NIH.[43]

Formal and informal communication is absolutely necessary to encourage technology transfer. But the perspectives of the two agencies are different: the NIH promotes and the FDA inhibits. With appropriate understanding, however, better cooperation could occur. There is evidence that such cooperation has developed in collaborative AIDS research. Perhaps because of the perceived crisis, and pressure on the FDA to behave as a promoter rather than as an inhibitor of AIDS activists, most observers have been impressed by the efforts of both federal agencies to cooperate.

The NIH and HCFA also interact. Because these agencies operate at different ends of the innovation spectrum, the interaction is rarely direct. However, an issue has arisen regarding NIH promotion of complex technologies such as the artificial heart. In the short term, and probably in the long term as well, the artificial heart will remain an extraordinarily expensive technology. The question is whether federal dollars should be spent developing a product that the federal government may never be able to provide to all the elderly that might benefit from it. Supporters argue that many scientific discoveries can be linked to the AHP program. Still others recognize that the research would never take place without federal support. Should there be controls on the promotion of potentially cost-increasing technologies, those very products that HCFA is trying to discourage? Does that smack of industrial policy or of federal domination of research for cost-control, rather than scientific, purposes?

Should the NIH promote cost-reducing technologies? Even if the marketplace has incentives for such products, would federal support give greater weight to their development, particularly to devices that could significantly reduce costs? One technology that has been suggested for federal attention is the development of devices to treat incontinence, an area where treatment has not yet made significant progress but which poses a major and expensive problem for the elderly. Urinary incontinence is the involuntary loss of urine severe enough to have social and/or hygienic consequences. It is a significant cause of disability and dependence. The monetary costs of management are conservatively estimated at $10.3 billion annually. The estimates are that at least ten million adult Americans suffer from incontinence to some degree, including half of all nursing home patients.[44]

Research is increasing the range of options, including medication, catheterization, urethral clamps, behavioral management, pelvic muscle exercises, implantation of an artificial urinary sphincter, electrotherapy, and surgery. Some therapies, such as collagen implants, cost over $1,800 for the kit, surely outside the price range of incontinent patients admitted to a long-term care facility. It may be that the marketplace already encourages innovation for cost-reducing technologies. However, one could argue that the NIH could be enlisted in the cost-containment war as well.

This section supplies a framework for thinking about the policy environment. Policy proliferation can lead to problems; these problems can be addressed by efforts to reconcile, reinforce, and coordinate interactions. These efforts require an understanding of the different missions of the policy institutions and the broad political context in which they operate.

10

THE FUTURE

A good part of the tribulations of patients (and
their physicians) comes from unreal attempts to
transcend the possible; to deny its limits, and to
seek the impossible: accommodation is more laborious and less exalted, and consists, in effect, of
a painstaking exploration of the full range of the
real and the possible.

Oliver Sacks
Awakenings

We have examined the patient, evaluated the prescriptions, and
considered modifications in the treatment.[1] Now is the time to
reflect on the prognosis. Prognostication is always problematic,
particularly so in the world of health. Wild cards can surprise
even the most meticulous diagnostician. There can be unexpected increases in demand for services. A few years ago, it is unlikely that anyone could have predicted the impact of the AIDS
epidemic on health care planning and services. Like Pearl Harbor, AIDS has precipitated a dramatic redefinition of priorities
and reallocation of resources. Supply can change as well. The
recent recognition that the United States has serious budgetary
problems and the growing recession of the early 1990s have
drastically increased pressures to limit health care expenditures.

Uncertainty in the health care marketplace is exacerbated by
unrealistic expectations. The compelling desire for good health
and a long life has led to excessive demands upon medicine and
medical technology. In the words of neurologist Oliver Sacks,
medicine is asked to "transcend the possible." Obviously, there
are limits to the power of machines. Despite what medical ethi-
cist Daniel Callahan has referred to as our "touching faith in

technical fixes," medical devices will never meet all the expectations imposed upon them.[2]

Without a realistic grasp of these limitations, we will be constantly disappointed. Unfortunately, dashed hopes create a tendency to blame devices for failing to live up to them. Just as medical technology cannot solve our battles with mortality, it cannot be held responsible for the failure to do so.

Similarly, the public needs to appreciate the dilemma facing innovators and manufacturers of medical products. These producers must respond to the economic realities of the private sector in which they operate. Manufacturers in a market economy try to expand their market share and make a profit. However, when a product is used for health care, the public traditionally has been uncomfortable with the consequences of the profit motive. Some have accused pharmaceutical companies of "unconscionable" profit. When the asking price exceeds what some customers (or some insurers) are willing or able to pay, is it unconscionable?

On the other hand, expansion of markets beyond what may be appropriate can have significant consequences for medical device consumers and the health care system as a whole. Adverse reactions to IUD implants in inappropriate candidates caused serious harm. In many respects, the traditional capitalist notions of markets can lead to socially irresponsible behavior. Supply-induced demand leads to waste and unnecessarily increases public and private expenditures.

Because of the value of these products and the expectations placed on their producers, public policy wrapped itself around the medical device industry. We must recall Lewis Mumford's wise words: "The machine itself makes no demands and holds out no promises; it is the human spirit that makes demands and keeps promises." Government policies and our public institutions must keep their promises. However, just as we have to learn to live with the limitations of technology, so we must understand the limitations of public policy in the United States.

Throughout this book, we have explored the dynamics of policy proliferation—the multiple, overlapping, often inconsistent interventions that reflect American history, political structure, and culture. Policy proliferation is inevitable in the American system of government. As Richard Neustadt, an astute observer of politics, has observed, we have not so much a government of separated powers as "a government of separated institutions sharing power."[3] Shared power has led to multiple interventions in its exercise, at both the federal and the state levels of government.

It is worth noting that shared power may offer benefits. For example, Justice Brandeis praised the states as "laboratories of experimentation." To some extent, our fragmented federal institutional structures may be laboratories as well. Experimentation implies distinctive solutions. Among these many alternatives, one of these laboratories of experimentation might get it right.

Tinkering with some unwanted effects of multiple public policies has been suggested in this book. Medical device innovators are tinkerers, and medical device policy benefits from the tinkerer's art. As was discussed in chapter 9, incremental adjustments can greatly improve the policy environment. Incremental reform involves, in Sacks's words, laborious, painstaking accommodations, no less important because they are less dramatic than sweeping structural changes.

Tinkering with policy processes, however, should not be the end of the story because it does not address the hard questions that society has yet to face. Callahan's point is well taken: changing the mechanics of the system is no substitute for examination of "the psychological, moral, and political assumptions that lie below it."[4] In the final analysis, the most important issues are neither questions of science and technology nor simple questions of policy reform. The underlying issues reflect moral values about how we want to live and how we want to die, as individuals and as a society. We need on-going discussions of moral values that concern equity, resource allocation, and responsibility for adverse outcomes, to name just a few. The controversy surrounding the state of Oregon's attempt to prioritize Medicaid services arose from our difficulty in facing challenging moral issues.

Medical device technology is integral to this moral debate. Indeed, consideration of the moral consequences has not kept pace with the ever-increasing capabilities of medical devices. Life-support equipment can keep human beings "alive" indefinitely, but is this artificial extension of life compelled by moral or ethical principles? Does the existence of the machine require its use? Should economic resources be relevant to these considerations?

Before the advent of life-extending technologies, these decisions were left to God or fate. Now, in whose hands do these decisions reside? Are they exclusively individual decisions for families and physicians? The substantial role of public institutions has raised many of these individual dilemmas to the realm of public policy. Government payers must allocate limited resources. Who should participate in these policy decisions: physicians, theologians, politicians, judges, patients?

Many policy institutions are restricted by their narrow jurisdictions. Thus, for example, we debate minor alterations of regulation of particular devices and whether to lower reimbursement to producers of home medical equipment. We seem to quibble at the margins without facing these larger questions. It is imperative that we find appropriate forums for debate. The halls of the Food and Drug Administration or the Health Care Financing Administration are not the proper places to do so. Congress and state legislatures could begin the process, although it is important that the debates rise above purely partisan politics. Additional forums must be created where the people who will have to live with these important decisions can participate and help work toward a consensus on pivotal questions.

Medical devices are critical weapons in the armamentarium against disease. As a society, we want to encourage the flow of new, effective innovations. However, the challenge is to promote sufficient and useful medical weaponry without encouraging a medical arms race. Overuse and misuse, as we have seen, induce excess demand, waste valuable resources, and may harm the very people the weapons are designed to protect.

We must manage this medical arms race. This book has told the story of "adroit inventions and adaptations in politics" and their consequences to the products, the producers, and the public. The system is not perfect; considerable work remains to be done. Our expectations of both the devices and the policies that affect them, however, must recognize their limitations. Only then can the painstaking exploration of the real and the possible succeed.

Notes

PREFACE

1. An excellent example is the recent work by Manuel Tratjenberg, *Economic Analysis of Product Innovation: The Case of CT Scanners* (Cambridge: Harvard University Press, 1990). In this work, the author uses the CT scan to quantify and analyze the notion of product innovation. However, he devotes only a scant four pages to the regulatory environment.

2. For work on the FDA, see Peter Temin, *Taking Your Medicine: Drug Regulation in the United States* (Cambridge: Harvard University Press, 1980); and Richard A. Merrill and Peter Barton Hutt, *Food and Drug Law* (Mineola, N.Y.: Foundation Press, 1980). For the National Institutes of Health, see Victoria A. Harden, *Inventing the NIH: Federal Biomedical Research Policy 1887–1937* (Baltimore: Johns Hopkins University Press, 1976); and Steven P. Strickland, *Politics, Science, and Dread Disease* (Cambridge: Harvard University Press, 1972). Louise B. Russell, *Medicare's New Hospital Payment System: Is It Working?* (Washington, D.C.: The Brookings Institution, 1989). These references are illustrative of the work in the field. More complete citations accompany the subsequent chapters.

3. Richard A. Rettig, "Lessons Learned from the End-Stage Renal Disease Experience," in R. H. Egdahl and Paul M. Gertman, eds., *Technology and the Quality of Health Care* (Germantown, Md.: Aspen Systems, 1978). Alonzo Plough, *Borrowed Time: Artificial Organs and the Politics of Extending Lives* (Philadelphia: Temple University Press, 1986). Natalie Davis Spingarn, *Heartbeat: The Politics of Health Research* (Washington, D.C.: Robert B. Luce, 1976).

4. U.S. Congress, Office of Technology Assessment, *Federal Policies and the Medical Devices Industry* (Washington, D.C.: GPO, October 1984) and *Medical Technology and the Costs of the Medicare Program* (Washington, D.C.: GPO, July 1984). Other government studies of importance, including reports and investigations by the General Accounting Office, are cited in subsequent chapters.

5. See, for example, Karen E. Ekelman, ed., *New Medical Devices: Factors Influencing Invention, Development, and Use* (Washington, D.C.: National Academy Press, 1988); and H. David Banta, "Major Issues

Facing Biomedical Innovation," in Edward B. Roberts, ed., *Biomedical Innovation* (Cambridge: MIT Press, 1981).

6. See, for example, Susan Bartlett Foote, "Loops and Loopholes: Hazardous Device Regulation under the 1976 Medical Device Amendments to the Food, Drug, and Cosmetics Act," *Ecology Law Quarterly* 7 (1978): 101–135; "Administrative Preemption: An Experiment in Regulatory Federalism," *Virginia Law Review* 70 (1984): 1429–1466; "From Crutches to CT Scans: Business-Government Relations and Medical Product Innovation," in James E. Post, ed., *Research in Corporate Social Performance and Policy* 8 (Greenwich, Conn.: JAI Press, 1986), 3–28; "Coexistence, Conflict, Cooperation: Public Policies toward Medical Devices," *Journal of Health Politics, Policy and Law* 11 (1986): 501–523; "Assessing Medical Technology Assessment: Past, Present, and Future," *Milbank Quarterly* 65 (1987): 59–80; "Product Liability and Medical Device Regulation: Proposal for Reform," in Karen E. Ekelman, ed., *New Medical Devices: Factors Influencing Invention, Development, and Use* (Washington, D.C.: National Academy Press, 1988), 73–92; and "Selling American Medical Equipment in Japan," *California Management Review* 31 (1989): 146–161.

7. Paul Starr, *The Social Transformation of American Medicine* (New York: Basic Books, 1982); Charles E. Rosenberg, *The Care of Strangers: The Rise of America's Hospital System* (New York: Basic Books, 1987); Rosemary Stevens, *In Sickness and in Wealth, American Hospitals in the Twenty-First Century* (New York: Basic Books, 1989); and Henry Grabowski and J. M. Vernon, *The Regulation of Pharmaceuticals: Balancing the Benefits and Risks* (Washington, D.C.: American Enterprise Institute, 1983). See also Grabowski, *Drug Regulation and Innovation: Empirical Evidence and Policy Options* (Washington, D.C.: American Enterprise Institute, 1976). The pharmaceutical industry has been well studied. See also Jonathan Liebernau, *Medical Science and Medical Industry: The Formation of the American Pharmaceutical Industry* (Baltimore: Johns Hopkins University Press, 1987).

CHAPTER 1

1. Lewis Mumford, *Technics and Civilization* (New York: Harcourt Brace Jovanovich, 1934).

2. Forecasts placed health care as rising from 11.9 percent of the GNP in 1990 to 13.1 percent in 1995. Alden Solovg, "Recession Prospects Mixed Bag for Health Care," cited in *Medical Benefits* 6 (30 August 1989).

3. Russell C. Coile, "Advances in the Next Decade Will Make To-

day's Technology Seem Primitive," cited in *Medical Benefits* 6 (30 August 1989).

4. Stanley Joel Reiser, *Medicine and the Reign of Technology* (Cambridge: Cambridge University Press, 1978).

5. The risks of the Bjork-Shiley heart valve, an implanted disk that controls the flow of blood through the heart, received publicity in 1990. The valve has a tendency to fail in some cases, leading to the deaths of recipients. The legal and regulatory issues raised by this medical device are discussed in chapter 6.

6. Cardiac pacemakers are discussed in chapters 4 and 5; intraocular lenses are studied in chapter 7.

7. See Karen Southwick, "Oregon Blazing a Trail with Plan to Ration Health Care," *Healthweek*, 12 March 1990, 30, 33. To implement its plan, Oregon needs waivers from some of the federal Medicaid requirements. In expanding coverage for poor families by restricting benefits, Oregon would violate a requirement that families receiving federal aid automatically receive full Medicaid coverage as well. Waivers can be granted administratively or through Congress. There is much political controversy about the rationing scheme. By the end of 1990, Oregon was revising its final priority list, and Congress was in a "wait-and-see" mode. Virginia Morell, "Oregon Puts Bold Health Plan on Ice," *Science* 249 (3 August 1990): 468–471.

8. An excellent study on the impact of policies on contraceptive research is Luigi Mastroianni, Jr., Peter J. Donaldson, and Thomas T. Kane, eds., *Developing New Contraceptives: Obstacles and Opportunities* (Washington, D.C.: National Academy Press, 1990).

9. Gordon C. Rausser, "Predatory Versus Productive Government: The Case of U.S. Agricultural Policies," *Journal of Economic Perspectives* 2 (Winter 1992).

10. Rausser defines some government policy as productive (reducing transaction costs and correcting market failures) and other policy as predatory (redistributing wealth without concern for growth or efficiency). His work seeks to explain and reconcile the perceived conflicts between the two approaches.

11. Congress protects the tobacco industry with a variety of favorable economic policies while simultaneously inhibiting the sale of tobacco products through television advertising limits and warning label requirements. Officials in several administrations have used their positions to condemn the marketing and the use of tobacco, and states and localities have severely restricted or banned smoking in public places.

12. The government protects the automobile industry with negotiated trade restrictions while also regulating automobile design to pro-

mote safety and environmental goals. Other federal policies regarding gasoline pricing and supply, highway construction, and alternative forms of transportation all affect the infrastructure upon which the automobile depends. The 1989 Alaskan oil spill revealed both redundancies and regulatory gaps between federal and state authorities and illustrated the problems that can arise when various government institutions impose overlapping or conflicting demands.

13. There is a vast literature on federalism. For an overview, see David B. Walker, *Toward a Functioning Federalism* (Cambridge, Mass.: Winthrop Publishers, 1981). For a discussion of federalism and health, see Frank J. Thompson, "New Federalism and Health Care Policy: States and the Old Questions," *Journal of Health Politics, Policy and Law* 11 (1986): 647–669.

14. 21 U.S.C. sec. 321(h). This definition appears in the 1976 Medical Device Amendments to the Food, Drug, and Cosmetic Act, discussed at great length in chapter 5.

15. The Office of Technology Assessment is a research arm of Congress and produces technical reports and evaluations at its request.

16. For a discussion of the history of the FDA, see chapter 2.

17. Foote, "From Crutches to CT Scans," 4.

18. Karl A. Fox, *Social Indicators* (New York: John Wiley, 1974).

19. Richard H. Shyrock, *American Medical Research, Past and Present* (New York: The Commonwealth Fund, 1947), 140.

20. Randall R. Bovbjerg, Philip J. Held, and Louis H. Diamond, "Provider-Patient Relations and Treatment Choice in an Era of Fiscal Incentives: The Case of the End-Stage Renal Disease Program," *Milbank Quarterly* 65 (1987): 177–202, 177.

21. In 1990, one dose of TPA cost $2,200, in contrast to the drug it claims to replace, streptokinase, which cost $200 a dose. U.S. sales of TPA in 1989 were nearly $200 million. Karen Southwick, "Analysts Say TPA Use May Drop in Wake of Study," *Healthweek*, 26 March, 1990, 45.

22. Grabowski and Vernon, *Regulation of Pharmaceuticals*, 18.

23. David J. Teece, "Profiting from Technological Innovation: Implications for Integration, Collaboration, Licensing, and Public Policy," *Research Policy* 15 (December 1986): 285–305.

24. For example, in *The Sources of Innovation* (New York: Oxford University Press, 1988), Eric von Hippel questions the assumption that manufacturers are the primary source of innovation. He presents studies to show that the sources of innovation vary greatly, often coming from the suppliers of component parts or the product users. He then develops a theory of the functional sources of innovation. In another recent work, *Economic Analysis of Product Innovation: The Case of*

CT Scanners (Cambridge: Harvard University Press, 1990), Manuel Trajtenberg presents a method to estimate the benefits from product innovations that accrue to the consumer over time, focusing particularly on the interaction between innovation and diffusion. For those interested in pursuing the study of innovation, see also Nathan Rosenberg, *Inside the Black Box: Technology and Economics* (Cambridge: Cambridge University Press, 1982); and Edwin Mansfield, *Industrial Research and Technological Innovation: An Econometric Analysis* (New York: Norton, 1968). For a thoughtful effort to identify the components of innovation, see James J. Zwolenik, *Science, Technology, and Innovation,* prepared for the National Science Foundation (Columbus, Ohio: Battelle Columbus Labs, February 1973).

25. John Jewkes et al., *The Sources of Innovation* (London: Macmillan, 1969).

26. Shyrock, *American Medical Research,* 2.

27. Jewkes, *Sources,* 28.

28. The literature emerges primarily from the fields of political science, history, and law. It is impossible to provide a complete bibliography, but a good place to start an inquiry on how government agencies work is James Q. Wilson, *Bureaucracy: What Government Agencies Do and Why They Do It* (New York: Basic Books, 1989) and his earlier book, *The Politics of Regulation* (New York: Basic Books, 1980). See also James O. Freedman, *Crisis and Legitimacy: The Administrative Process and American Government* (Cambridge: Cambridge University Press, 1978). For discussion of how bureaucrats make decisions, see Eugene Bardach and Robert Kagan, *Going By the Book: The Problem of Regulatory Unreasonableness* (Philadelphia: Temple University Press, 1982); and Graham Allison, *Essence of Decision* (Boston: Little, Brown, 1971). For an understanding of the legislative process, begin with Eric Redman, *The Dance of Legislation* (New York: Simon and Schuster, 1973); and Hedrick Smith, *The Power Game* (New York: McGraw-Hill, 1988). For introduction to the judiciary, see Robert A. Carp and Ronald Stidham, *Judicial Process in America* (Washington, D.C.: Congressional Quarterly Press, 1990). For a discussion of litigation, see Jethro K. Lieberman, *The Litigious Society* (New York: Basic Books, 1981).

29. For an excellent discussion of values in relation to public policy, see generally William W. Lowrance, *Modern Science and Human Values* (New York: Oxford University Press, 1985).

30. U.S. Department of Commerce, Bureau of the Census, *Statistical Abstract of the United States, 1985* (Washington, D.C.: GPO, 1984), table 143.

31. U.S. Congress, Office of Technology Assessment, *Federal Policies*

and the Medical Devices Industry (Washington, D.C.: GPO, October 1984).

32. Preamble to Medical Devices Amendment, Public Law 94–295, 90 Stat. 539.

CHAPTER 2

1. Russell Baker, *Growing Up* (New York: New American Library, 1982), 36–38.

2. Stephen Toulmin, "Technological Progress and Social Policy: The Broader Significance of Medical Mishaps," in Mark Siegler et al., eds., *Medical Innovation and Bad Outcomes: Legal, Social, and Ethical Responses* (Ann Arbor: Health Administration Press, 1987), 22.

3. Selma J. Mushkin, Lynn C. Paringer, and Milton M. Chen, "Returns to Biomedical Research, 1900–1975: An Initial Assessment of Impacts on Health Expenditures," in Richard H. Egdahl and Paul M. Gertman, eds., *Technology and the Quality of Health Care* (Germantown, Md.: Aspen Systems, 1978).

4. Charles E. Rosenberg, *Caring for Strangers: The Rise of America's Hospital System* (New York: Basic Books, 1987). This is a comprehensive study of American hospitals from 1800 to 1920.

5. Richard H. Shyrock, *American Medical Research, Past and Present* (New York: The Commonwealth Fund, 1947).

6. Ibid., 99.

7. Paul Starr, *The Social Transformation of American Medicine* (New York: Basic Books, 1982), 79–145. This comprehensive study of American medical practice is a classic.

8. Leonard S. Reich, *The Making of American Industrial Research: Science and Business at GE and Bell, 1876–1926* (Cambridge: Cambridge University Press, 1985), 24.

9. Ibid., 240.

10. John P. Swann, *American Scientists and the Pharmaceutical Industry: Cooperative Research in Twentieth-Century America* (Baltimore: Johns Hopkins University Press, 1988).

11. Shyrock, *American Medical Research*, 145.

12. The debate about the appropriate role of academic scientists within universities and about private sector profits continues to this day. For a discussion of the current debate and the relevant public policy on these issues, see chapter 3.

13. Shyrock, *American Medical Research*, 143.

14. Ibid., 122.

15. Chevalier Jackson, *The Life of Chevalier Jackson: An Autobiography* (New York: Macmillan, 1938), 197.

16. Department of Commerce, Bureau of the Census, *Historical Statistics of the United States, Colonial Times to 1970,* bicentennial edition, pt. 2, ser. 221, 247 (Washington, D.C.: GPO, 1975).

17. Reich, *American Industrial Research,* 89, citing George Wise, *The Corporations' Chemist* (Unpublished manuscript, 1981), 237.

18. Most of the information on Arnold Beckman and the founding of his company appears in Harrison Stephens, *Golden Past, Golden Future: The First Fifty Years of Beckman Instruments, Inc.* (Claremont, Calif.: Claremont University Center, 1985).

19. Stephens, *Golden Past,* 14.

20. Much of the history of Arnold Beckman's contributions were summarized in Carol Moberg, ed., *The Beckman Symposium on Biomedical Instrumentation* (New York: Rockefeller University, 1986). This volume celebrates the fiftieth anniversary of the founding of Beckman Instruments.

21. Reich, *American Industrial Research,* 3.

22. Ibid., 37.

23. Kendall Birr, *Pioneering in Industrial Research: The Story of the General Electric Research Laboratory* (Washington, D.C.: Public Affairs Press, 1957).

24. The government's role in World War I represents the beginning of a transition to government involvement in medical device innovation. In this case, the government's demand for X-ray equipment as a purchaser significantly benefited the firm.

25. The term *quack* dates to the sixteenth century and is an abbreviation for *quacksalver.* The term refers to a charlatan who brags or "quacks" about the curative or "salving" powers of the product without knowing anything about medical care. From the *Washington Post,* 8 July 1985, 6.

26. Warren E. Schaller and Charles R. Carroll, *Health Quackery and the Consumer* (Philadelphia: W. B. Saunders, 1976), 228. This volume contains many descriptions of a variety of fraudulent devices. It makes for amusing reading, but deceptive activities left a lasting legacy on the medical device industry.

27. James H. Young, *Medical Messiahs* (Princeton: Princeton University Press, 1967), 243.

28. Ibid.

29. Schaller and Carroll, *Health Quackery,* 226.

30. Drown v. U.S., 198 F.2d 999 (1952). Drown was prosecuted for grand larceny and died while awaiting trial. See Joseph Cramp, ed.,

Nostrums and Quackery and Pseudo-Medicine, vols. 1–3 (Chicago: Press of the American Medical Association).

31. Concern about fraudulent drugs and devices surfaces periodically. Congress has held hearings investigating health frauds, particularly frauds against the elderly. See, for example, House Select Committee on Aging, *Frauds Against the Elderly: Health Quackery,* 96th Cong., 2d sess., no. 96–251 (Washington, D.C.: GPO, 1980). In 1984, the FDA devoted only about one-half of 1 percent of its budget to fighting quack products. Under pressure from the outside, it set up a fraud branch in 1985 to process enforcement actions. See Don Colburn, "Quackery: Medical Fraud Is Proliferating and the FDA Can't Seem to Stop It," *Washington Post National Weekly Edition,* 8 July 1985, 6. For a description of past and present device quackery, see Stephen Barrett and Gilda Knight, eds., *The Health Robbers: How to Protect Your Money and Your Life* (Philadelphia: George F. Stickley, 1976).

32. In addition to the extensive data gathered by the Census, see R. D. Peterson and C. R. MacPhee, *Economic Organization in Medical Equipment and Supply* (Lexington, Mass.: D. C. Heath, 1973).

33. Shyrock, *American Medical Research,* 77.

34. Quoted in Harden, *Inventing the NIH,* 3.

35. Ibid., 92.

36. Ibid., 28.

37. Ibid., 93.

38. Ibid., 127.

39. Ibid., 132.

40. Ibid., 91.

41. For a thorough discussion of the politics of the NIH's role in cancer research, see Richard A. Rettig, *A Cancer Crusade: The Story of the National Cancer Act of 1971* (Princeton: Princeton University Press, 1977).

42. Shyrock, *American Medical Research,* 78–79.

43. Oscar E. Anderson, "Pioneer Statute: The Pure Food and Drug Act of 1906," *Journal of Public Law* 13 (1964): 189–196. See also Oscar E. Anderson, *The Health of a Nation: Harvey W. Wiley and the Fight for Pure Food* (Chicago: University of Chicago Press, 1958).

44. Thomas A. Bailey, "Congressional Opposition to the Pure Food Legislation, 1879–1906," *American Journal of Sociology* 36 (July 1930): 52–64.

45. Ibid.

46. Since 1820, the United States Pharmacopeia Convention (USPC) has set standards for medications used by the American public. It is an independent, nonprofit corporation composed of delegates

from colleges of medicine and pharmacy, state medical associations, and other national associations concerned with medicine. When Congress passed the first major drug safety law in 1906, the standards recognized in the statute were those of the USPC. Its major publication, the *United States Pharmacopeia* (*USP*), is the world's oldest regularly revised national compendium. Today it continues to be the official compendia for standards for drugs.

47. Proprietary drugs are those drugs sold directly to the public, and they include patent medicines. The term *proprietary* indicates that the ingredients are secret, not that they are patented.

48. Temin, *Taking Your Medicine*, 28.

49. Pure Food Act, 34 Stat. 674 (1906).

50. A. Hunter Dupree, *Science in the Federal Government: A History of Policies and Activities to 1940* (Cambridge: Harvard University Press, 1957), 179.

51. Bruce C. Davidson, "Preventive 'Medicine' for Medical Devices: Further Regulation Required?" *Marquette Law Review* 55 (Fall 1972): 408–455.

52. Temin, *Taking Your Medicine*, 38.

53. U.S. Department of Agriculture, *Report of the Chief of the Food and Drug Administration* (Washington, D.C.: GPO, 1933), 13–14.

54. Davidson, "Preventive 'Medicine,'" 414.

55. Ibid., 415.

56. Temin, *Taking Your Medicine*, 42.

57. 21 U.S.C. sec. 351–352.

58. See Comptroller General of the United States, *Lack of Authority Limits Consumer Protection: Problems in Identifying and Removing from the Market Products Which Violate the Law,* B–164031(2) at 18–25 (1972).

59. See Rosenberg, *Caring for Strangers*.

60. Starr, *Transformation*, 148–180.

61. Ibid., 237. Starr attributes European activity to political instability not present in the United States. The American government remained very decentralized, and there was not the political instability that Europe encountered.

62. Ibid., 245–253.

63. Ibid., 340.

64. Harvey Brooks, "National Science Policy and Technological Innovation," in Ralph Landau and Nathan Rosenberg, eds., *The Positive Sum Strategy: Harnessing Technology for Economic Growth* (Washington, D.C.: National Academy Press, 1986), 119–167, 123.

65. Stephens, *Golden Past*, 34.

66. This information comes from Baxter Travenol Laboratories

Public Relations Department. The publication is entitled "The History of Baxter Travenol" and is unpaginated.

67. John Anderson Miller, *Men and Volts at War: The Story of General Electric in World War II* (New York: McGraw-Hill, 1947).

68. Ibid., 11.

69. Ibid., 189.

CHAPTER 3

1. Since 1960, federal funds have accounted for from 47 to 66 percent of all R&D spending in the United States. There are three trends in federal support: (1) from the late 1940s to about 1967 there was steady growth in all areas, with 1957 being a starting point for the NIH budget; (2) from 1967 to 1977 there was a general leveling off of investment in space and defense, although life sciences held steady; and (3) from 1977 and throughout the Reagan era defense spending increased at the expense of civilian R&D. Harvey Brooks, "National Science Policy and Technological Innovation," in Landau and Rosenberg, eds., *The Positive Sum Strategy*. Overall, defense related R&D accounted for about 50 to 60 percent of total federal expenditures throughout the period. See discussion in Richard M. Cyert and David C. Mowery, eds., *Technology and Employment: Innovation and Growth in the U.S. Economy* (Washington, D.C.: National Academy Press, 1987), 35–38.

2. James A. Shannon, "Advancement of Medical Research: A Twenty-Year View of the Role of the National Institutes of Health," *Journal of Medical Education* 42 (1967): 97–108, 98.

3. Cited in Natalie Davis Spingarn, *Heartbeat: The Politics of Health Research* (Washington, D.C.: Robert B. Luce, 1976), 28.

4. Shannon, "Advancement," 100.

5. Spingarn, *Heartbeat*, 25.

6. Cited in Shannon, "Advancement," 101.

7. Spingarn, *Heartbeat*, 2.

8. Ruth S. Hanft, "Biomedical Research: Influence on Technology," in R. Southby et al., eds., *Health Care Technology Under Financial Constraints* (Columbus, Ohio: Battelle Press, 1987), 160–171, 167.

9. U.S. Department of Health and Human Services, *Abstracts of Small Business Innovation Research (SBIR) Phase I and Phase II Projects, Fiscal Year 1987*. Under the SBIR, phase I awards are generally for $50,000 for a period of about six months and are intended for technical feasibility studies. Phase II, for periods of one to three years, continues the research effort initiated in phase I, and awards do not

exceed $500,000. In 1987, NIH awards to the SBIR accounted for $61.6 million.

10. Senate Committee on Appropriations, Subcommittee on Labor, Health and Human Services, Education and Related Agencies, *NIH Budget Request for Fiscal Year 1989,* cited in testimony of Frank E. Samuel, Jr., president, Health Industry Manufacturers Association (Unpublished document from HIMA, 24 May 1988).

11. Julius H. Comroe, Jr., and Robert D. Dripps, "Scientific Basis for the Support of Biomedical Science," *Science* 192 (April 1976): 105–111.

12. Brooks, "National Science Policy," 122, citing Philip Handler, ed., *The Life Sciences* (Washington, D.C.: National Academy of Sciences, 1970); and Henry G. Grabowski and John M. Vernon, "The Pharmaceutical Industry," in Richard R. Nelson, ed., *Government and Technical Progress: A Cross-Industry Analysis* (New York: Pergamon Press, 1982), 283–360.

13. Engineering Research Board, "Bioengineering Systems Research in the United States: An Overview," in *Directions in Engineering Research: An Assessment of Opportunities and Needs* (Washington, D.C.: National Academy Press, 1987), 77–112, 79. While it is true that the National Science Foundation (NSF) sponsors projects in scientific and engineering research, many of which are in biological engineering, the resources of the NSF are significantly less than those of the NIH. For example, in fiscal year 1988, funding for molecular biosciences at NSF was $44.6 million, for cellular biosciences, $54.24 million, and for instrumentation and resources, $34.15 million. *National Science Foundation, Guide to Programs, Fiscal Year 1989* (Washington, D.C.: GPO, 1989). Compare this to the 1986 budget of the National Heart, Lung, and Blood Institute, only one of the institutes within the NIH, which received $821,901,000 for fiscal year 1986. *National Heart, Lung, and Blood Institute, Fact Book, Fiscal Year 1986* (Washington, D.C.: GPO, 1986).

14. Cited in Spingarn, *Heartbeat,* 32.

15. This book focuses on the artificial heart program. For more extensive discussion of the War on Cancer, see Rettig, *A Cancer Crusade;* for kidney dialysis, see Plough, *Borrowed Time;* and Renee C. Fox and Judith P. Swazey, *The Courage to Fail: A Social View of Organ Transplants and Dialysis,* 2d ed. (Chicago: University of Chicago Press, 1973). Dialysis is discussed at greater length in chapter 4.

16. As more was learned about the complexities of the technology, the numbers have been revised dramatically downward. See Working Group on Mechanical Circulatory Support of the National Heart,

Lung, and Blood Institute, *Artificial Heart and Assist Devices: Directions, Needs, Costs, Societal and Ethical Issues* (May 1985), 16.

17. Ibid., 9–14.

18. *New York Times,* 17 May 1988, B7.

19. This involvement was later institutionalized in the Small Business Innovation Development Act of 1982, which increased the role of small businesses in federally supported research and development (Public Law 97–219). This law created the Small Business Innovation Research (SBIR) Program, involving eleven federal agencies, of which the Department of Health and Human Services (HHS) is the second largest participant. The NIH accounts for 92 percent of the SBIR activity in the DHHS. The goal is to support the small business through early stages of research so that it can attract private capital and commercialize the results. U.S. Department of Health and Human Services, *Abstracts of SBIR Projects, Fiscal Year 1987.*

20. One of the successful contractors, Novacor, a small, innovative company, is profiled in chapter 9.

21. Spingarn, *Heartbeat,* 148.

22. Ibid., 152.

23. *New York Times,* 8 July 1988.

24. See discussion in Eugene M. Emme, *Aeronautics and Astronautics: An American Chronology of Science and Technology in the Exploration of Space, 1915–1960* (Washington, D.C.: NASA, 1961), 87.

25. Jane van Nimmen and Leonard C. Bruno, eds., *NASA Historical Data Book* (Washington, D.C.: NASA, 1988), 6.

26. NASA Center History Series, *Adventures in Research* (Washington, D.C.: NASA, 1970), 370.

27. Van Nimmen and Bruno, *Historical Data Book,* 244.

28. NASA, *SpinOFF* (Washington, D.C.: NASA, 1958), 3. *SpinOFF,* an annual NASA publication, describes technologies that have been produced using NASA expertise. The examples that appear in the text were derived from a review of *SpinOFF* stories.

29. NASA, *SpinOFF* (1984), 61.

30. NASA, *SpinOFF* (1985), 25.

31. NASA, *SpinOFF* (1987), 76–77.

32. NASA, *SpinOFF* (1983), 88.

33. NASA, *SpinOFF* (1981), 74–75.

34. NASA, *SpinOFF* (1981), 88–91.

35. For a complete history of ultrasound, see Barry B. Goldberg and Barbara A. Kimmelman, eds., *Medical Diagnostic Ultrasound: A Retrospective on Its Fortieth Anniversary* (Rochester, N.Y.: Eastman Kodak

Company, 1988), 3; this book also contains an extensive list of references.

36. Frost & Sullivan, *Ultrasonic Medical Market* (New York: June 1975); Frost & Sullivan, *Government Sponsored Medical Instrumentation, Device and Diagnostics Research and Development* (New York: March 1978). Cited and discussed in William G. Mitchell, "Dynamic Commercialization: An Organizational Economic Analysis of Innovation in the Medical Diagnostic Imaging Industry" (Unpublished dissertation, School of Business Administration, University of California, Berkeley, 1988).

37. Mitchell, "Dynamic Commercialization," fig. 4.3.

38. U.S. Congress, Office of Technology Assessment, *The Maturation of Laser Technology: Social and Technical Factors*, prepared under contract to the Laser Institute of America by Joan Lisa Bromberg, Contract No. H3–5210, January 1988.

39. Bromberg, "Lasers," 28.

40. *The Implications of Reduced Defense Demand for the Electronics Industry, U.S. Arms Control, and Disarmament Agency* (Columbus, Ohio: Battelle Memorial Institute, September 1965), cited in Bromberg, "Lasers," 33.

41. *Biomedical Business International* 10:12 (14 July 1987): 113–115.

42. "Now Lasers Are Taking Aim at Heart Disease," *Business Week,* 19 December 1988, 98.

43. Cyert and Mowery, *Technology,* 37, citing Richard Nelson and R. Langlois, "Industrial Innovation Policy: Lessons from American History," *Science* 217 (February 1983): 814–818.

44. Ibid., citing Leslie Brueckner and Michael Borrus, "Assessing the Commercial Impact of the VHSIC Program" (Paper delivered at the Berkeley Roundtable on the International Economy, University of California, Berkeley, 1984).

45. John P. Swann, *American Scientists and the Pharmaceutical Industry* (Baltimore: Johns Hopkins University Press, 1988), 170.

46. Mitchell, "Dynamic Commercialization," 107.

47. Adeline B. Hale and Arthur B. Hale, eds., *Medical and Healthcare Marketplace Guide* (Miami: International Biomedical Information Service, 1986).

48. The term *diagnostic imaging* refers to medical technologies such as X-ray and magnetic resonance imaging (MRI and ultrasound, among others).

49. Mitchell, "Dynamic Commercialization," chap. 5.

50. Cited in Calvin Sims, "Business-Campus Ventures Grow," *New York Times,* 14 December 1987, 25, 27. The top university recipients in

1986 were Massachusetts Institute of Technology, Georgia Institute of Technology, Carnegie Mellon University, Pennsylvania State University, and University of Washington.

51. Judith Nowak, "The University of Michigan Policy Environment for University-Industry Interaction" (Paper delivered at Institute of Medicine Workshop on Government-Industry Collaboration in Biomedical Research and Education, Washington, D.C., 26–29 February, 1989).

52. David Blake, remarks at the Institute of Medicine, Forum on Drug Development and Regulation, Washington, D.C., 3 March 1989.

53. Public Law 96–517 (12 December 1980).

54. Public Law 98–620 (9 October 1984).

55. Mitchell, "Dynamic Commercialization," 110.

56. Public Law 96–480 (October 1980).

57. Public Law 99–953 (1986).

58. Executive Order 12591, *Facilitating Access to Science and Technology* (April 1987).

59. Brooks, "National Science Policy," 155.

CHAPTER 4

1. For data on spending, see R. M. Gibson et al., "National Health Expenditures, 1982," *Health Care Financing Review* 9 (Fall 1987): 23–24. See also Daniel R. Waldo et al., "National Health Expenditures, 1985," *Health Care Financing Review* 8 (Fall 1986).

2. Commission on Hospital Care, *Hospital Care in the United States: A Study of the Function of the General Hospital, Its Role in the Care of All Types of Illnesses, and the Conduct of Activities Related to Patient Service with Recommendations for Its Extension and Integration for More Adequate Care of the American Public* (New York: The Commonwealth Fund, 1947).

3. Public Law 79–725. For a complete description of the history of the Hill-Burton Program, see Judith R. Lave and Lester B. Lave, *The Hospital Construction Act: An Evaluation of the Hill-Burton Program, 1948–1973* (Washington, D.C.: American Enterprise Institute, 1974).

4. Lave and Lave, *Hospital Construction,* chap. 1.

5. Ibid., 25.

6. Ibid., 37.

7. Starr, *Transformation,* 286.

8. Arthur J. Altmeyer, *The Formative Years of Social Security* (Madison: University of Wisconsin Press, 1968), 185–186, cited in Starr, *Transformation,* 286 n. 151.

9. Starr, *Transformation*, 289.

10. Foote, "Crutches to CT Scans," 10.

11. Quoted in Andrew Stein, "Medicare's Broken Promises," *New York Times Magazine*, 17 February 1985, 44, 84. For a detailed discussion of the politics of Medicare, see Starr, *Transformation*, book. 2, chap. 1; see also Rashi Fein, *Medical Care, Medical Costs: The Search for a Health Insurance Policy* (Cambridge: Harvard University Press, 1986).

12. These changes, which altered the thrust of the program, are discussed in chapter 7 along with other cost-containment policies.

13. Social Security Amendments of 1972, Public Law 92–603. The specific impact of this legislation on kidney dialysis equipment is discussed in the next section of this chapter.

14. U.S. Congress, Office of Technology Assessment, *Medical Technology and the Costs of the Medicare Program* (Washington, D.C.: GPO, July 1984), 3.

15. See Waldo et al., "National Health Expenditures."

16. Lave and Lave, *Hospital Construction*, 54.

17. U.S. Department of Health and Human Services, *1987 budget request*, 5 February 1986.

18. National Advisory Council on Health Care Technology Assessment, *The Medicare Coverage Process* (14 September 1988). This report reviews and then critiques HCFA's coverage process.

19. For detailed discussion of OHTA, see Committee for Evaluating Medical Technologies in Clinical Use, *Assessing Medical Technologies* (Washington, D.C.: National Academy Press, 1985), particularly 355–363.

20. For a complete description of the Medicaid program, see Allen D. Spiegel, ed., *The Medicaid Experience* (Germantown, Md.: Aspen Systems, 1979). See also Thomas W. Grannemann and Mark V. Pauly, *Controlling Medicaid Costs: Federalism, Competition, and Choice* (Washington, D.C.: American Enterprise Institute, 1982); and Robert Stevens and Rosemary Stevens, *Welfare Medicine in America: A Case of Medicaid* (New York: Free Press, 1974).

21. Stephen F. Loebs, "Medicaid: A Survey of Indicators and Issues," in Spiegel, *The Medicaid Experience*, 5–19.

22. Charles N. Oberg and Cynthia Longseth Polich, "Medicaid: Entering the Third Decade," *Health Affairs* 7 (Fall 1988): 83–96, 85.

23. Loebs, "Medicaid," 6–8.

24. U.S. Bureau of the Census, *Census of Manufactures: Industry Series* (Washington, D.C.: GPO, 1963, 1982), table 6c.

25. Janice M. Cauwels, *The Body Shop: Bionic Revolutions in Medicine* (St. Louis: C. V. Mosby, 1986), chap. 12. For additional discussion of

dialysis, see B. D. Colen, *Hard Choices: Mixed Blessings of Modern Medical Technology* (New York: Putnam, 1986).

26. Rettig, "Lessons Learned," 154.

27. Ibid., 154–156.

28. David Sanders and Jesse Dukeninier, Jr., "Medical Advance and Legal Lag: Hemodialysis and Kidney Transplantation," *UCLA Law Review* 15 (1968): 357–413, 366.

29. Rettig, "Lessons Learned," 161–162, citing discussion in *Biomedical Engineering Development and Production,* a report by the Biomedical Engineering Resource Corporation, State of Illinois, to the National Institute of General Medical Sciences, National Institutes of Health, Washington, D.C. (July 1969), 12–21. See also National Academy of Engineering, Committee on the Interplay of Engineering with Biology and Medicine, *Government Patent Policy* (Washington, D.C.: National Academy of Engineering, 1970).

30. See, generally, Plough, *Borrowed Time.*

31. U.S. Congress, Office of Technology Assessment, "Medical Technology," 34–36.

32. John C. Moskop, "The Moral Limits to Federal Funding for Kidney Disease," *Hastings Center Report* (April 1987): 11–15.

33. Plough, *Borrowed Time,* 128–129.

34. Ibid., 130–154.

35. Ibid., 137.

36. Moskop, responding to letters criticizing his article "Moral Limits," in *Hastings Center Report* (December 1987): 43–44. See also the letters of Gerald H. Dessner and Carole Robbins Myers on pp. 42–43 of the same issue.

37. For a discussion of the comparative benefits of imaging technologies, see Mitchell, "Dynamic Commercialization," chap. 4, 42–56.

38. Bruce J. Hillman, "Government Health Policy and the Diffusion of New Medical Devices," *Health Services Research* 21 (December 1986): 681–711, 689.

39. U.S. Congress, Office of Technology Assessment, *Policy Implications of the Computed Tomography (CT) Scanner* (Washington, D.C.: GPO, August 1978).

40. Earl P. Steinberg, Jane E. Sisk, and Katherine E. Locke, "X-ray CT and Magnetic Resonance Imagers: Diffusion Patterns and Policy Issues," *New England Journal of Medicine* 313 (3 October 1985): 859–864, 860.

41. Data on sales in the industry are available from *Diagnostic Imaging* (San Francisco: Miller-Freeman Publishing, 1979–1990).

42. *Diagnostic Imaging* (1981), 2. Annual sales data for 1981.

43. Alan L. Hillman and J. Sanford Schwartz, "The Adoption and Diffusion of CT and MRI in the United States: A Comparative Analysis," *Medical Care* 23 (November 1985): 1283–1294, 1288.

44. The early cost-containment policies, including Certificate of Need (CON) and state based efforts to limit diffusion, will be discussed in detail in chapter 7. It is worth noting that we have begun to see the impact of policy proliferation as conflicting policies arise. At this point, however, cost-containment plans were relatively ineffective and diffusion proceeded apace.

45. Hillman, "Government Health Policy," 691–692.

46. See Hillman, "Government Health Policy"; Hillman and Schwartz, "Adoption and Diffusion"; and Steinberg et al., "X-ray CT."

47. Battelle Columbus Laboratories, "Interactions of Science and Technology in the Innovative Process: Some Case Studies," report prepared for the National Science Foundation, Contract NSF–C 667 (Columbus, Ohio: 19 March 1973), see sec. 5, 1–14.

48. Wilson Greatbatch, "Vignette 8: The First Successful Implantable Cardiac Pacemaker," in U.S. Office of Technology Assessment, *Inventors' Vignettes: Success and Failure in the Development of Medical Devices,* Contractors' Documents, Health Program (Washington, D.C., October 1986), 8:1–15.

49. Ibid., 8:5.

50. *Biomedical Business International* 10 (14 September 1987): 136–137.

51. Ibid. See also Robert McGough, "Everybody's Money," *Forbes,* 27 February 1984, 149, 152.

52. *Biomedical Business International* 10 (14 September 1987): 137.

53. Ibid.

54. Medicare payments in 1984 totaled $42 billion to 6,000 hospitals. Sales apparently fell off slightly in response to reimbursement and pricing pressures in the next two years. By 1986 the market resumed growth, with forecasts of 6 percent per unit and 10 percent revenue growth per year between 1987 and 1990.

55. Kidder, Peabody, "Cardiac Pacemaker Industry Analysis, 22 January 1981," cited in the Office of Inspector General, Draft Audit Report, *More Efficient Procurement of Heart Pacemakers Could Result in Medicare Savings of Over $64 Million Annually,* ACN 08–22608, submitted to the Senate Special Committee on Aging, *Hearings on Fraud, Waste, and Abuse in the Medicare Pacemaker Industry,* 97th Cong., 2d sess. (Washington, D.C.: GPO, 1982), 139–140.

56. *Hearings on Fraud, Waste, and Abuse,* app. 2, item 6, Draft Audit

Report, HHS, 2 September 1982, from Richard P. Kusserow, inspector general, to Carolyne Davis, administrator, HCFA.

57. *Hearings on Fraud, Waste, and Abuse*, testimony of Howard Hofferman, 30–50.

58. Comptroller General, Report to the Chair, Senate Special Committee on Aging, *Medicare's Policies and Prospective Payment Rates for Cardiac Pacemaker Surgeries Need Review and Revision*, GAO–HRD–85–39, 26 February 1985.

59. Senate Special Committee on Aging, *Pacemakers Revisited: A Saga of Benign Neglect*, 99th Cong., 1st sess. (Washington, D.C.: GPO, 1985), 99–104, 129.

60. Michael Allen, "Cordis Admits It Hid Defects of Pacemakers," *Wall Street Journal*, 1 September 1988, 6.

61. *Washington Post*, 13 August 1989, 41.

62. "Medtronic Inc. Expects Record Sales and Profit in Current Fiscal Year," *Wall Street Journal*, 21 August 1987, 6.

CHAPTER 5

1. House Committee on Government Operations, *Hearings on Regulation of Medical Devices (Intrauterine Contraceptive Devices)*, 93rd Cong., 1st sess. (Washington, D.C.: GPO, 1973), 180.

2. Davidson, "Preventive 'Medicine' for Medical Devices: Is Further Regulation Required?" *Marquette Law Review* 55 (Fall 1972): 423–424.

3. Milstead, *1963 Congress on Quackery*, 30.

4. Ibid.

5. Temin, *Taking Your Medicine*, 123–126.

6. See discussion in chapter 2.

7. U.S. Department of Health, Education, and Welfare, Cooper Committee, *Medical Devices: A Legislative Plan, Study Group on Medical Devices* (Washington, D.C.: GPO, 1970). Cited and discussed in *Medical Device Amendments of 1975, Hearings on H.R. 5545, H.R. 974, and S. 510 Before the Subcommittee on Health and the Environment of the Committee on Interstate and Foreign Commerce*, statement of Rep. Fred B. Rooney, 94th Cong., 1st sess., 199. See also Theodore Cooper, "Device Legislation," *Food, Drug, Cosmetic Law Journal* 26 (April 1971): 165–172. There have been challenges to the data in the Cooper report, but the public attention the study received made the issue of device safety politically salient.

8. U.S. Comptroller General, *Food and Drug Administration's Investigation of Defective Cardiac Pacemakers Recalled by the General Electric Company* 21 (1975). GE decided to voluntarily recall over 22,000 pace-

makers because some malfunctioned due to moisture that seeped into the pacemaker circuitry, probably due to faulty seals.

9. See discussion in this section.

10. 389 F.2d 825 (2d Cir. 1968).

11. 394 U.S. 784 (1969).

12. 25 *Federal Register* 9370 (30 September 1960).

13. 394 U.S. 784, 798 (1969).

14. The Dalkon Shield claimed to be superior to other products because of its unique shape. The nature of the product and the harms related to its design are discussed more fully in chapter 6.

15. *House Hearings on Medical Devices,* Advisory Committee on Obstetrics and Gynecology of the Food and Drug Administration, *Report on Intrauterine Contraceptive Devices* (1968), 441.

16. *House Hearings on Regulation of Medical Devices,* memorandum of William Goodrich, assistant general counsel of the FDA, 19 March 1968, 205–206.

17. 44 *Federal Register* 6173 (31 January 1979).

18. *House Hearings on Regulation of Medical Devices,* 183.

19. *House Hearings on Regulation of Medical Devices,* statement of Peter Barton Hutt, 209.

20. Enter policy proliferation. The company's action may well have been motivated primarily by the fear of lawsuits, not the fear of FDA action. In any event, the FDA had few powers to invoke. Issues relating to product liability will be discussed in chapter 6.

21. Pacemaker hearings, medical device (IUD) hearings.

22. Public Law 94–295, 90 Stat. 539 (1976) codified at 21 United States Code secs. 360c–360k (1982), (a)(1–3). For detailed discussion of the Medical Device Amendments, see Foote, "Loops and Loopholes"; David A. Kessler, Stuart M. Pape, and David N. Sundwall, "The Federal Regulation of Medical Devices," *New England Journal of Medicine* 317 (6 August 1987): 357–366; and Jonathan S. Kahan, "The Evolution of FDA Regulation of New Medical Device Technology and Product Applications," *Food, Drug, Cosmetic Law Journal* 41 (1986): 207–214.

23. See letter from Representative Paul Rogers, one of the authors of the legislation to Alexander Schmidt, commissioner of the FDA, 21 June 1976 (cited in Foote, "Administrative Preemption," 1446, n. 74).

24. The process is referred to as a 510k after the number of the provision in the bill.

25. For example, Report of the House Subcommittee on Oversight and Investigations, Committee on Energy and Commerce, *Medical*

Device Regulation: The FDA's Neglected Child (Washington, D.C.: GPO, 1983); Comptroller General Report to Congress, *Federal Regulation of Medical Devices—Problems Still to Be Overcome,* GAO–HRD–83–53 (Washington, D.C.: General Accounting Office, September 1983); United States General Accounting Office, Report to the Chairman, Senate Committee on Governmental Affairs, *Early Warning of Problems Is Hampered by Severe Underreporting,* GAO–PEMD–87–1 (Washington, D.C.: General Accounting Office, December 1986); and General Accounting Office, Briefing Report to the Chairman, House Subcommittee on Health and the Environment, Committee on Energy and Commerce, *Medical Device Recalls: An Overview and Analysis 1983–1988,* GAO–PEMD–89–15r (Washington, D.C.: General Accounting Office, August 1989).

26. 766 F.2d 592 (1985).

27. 21 U.S.C. sec. 360j(1)(1)(E).

28. 48 *Federal Register* 56, 778 (1983).

29. General Medical v. FDA, 770 F.2d 214 (1985).

30. The device is used to electrically stimulate the cerebellar cortex of a patient's brain in treatment of intractable epilepsy and some movement disorders.

31. *Medical Device Bulletin* (Washington, D.C.: FDA, August 1984). See also Kessler et al., "Federal Regulation," 362, nn. 5, 12.

32. The excessive detail in the law derives from a congressional desire to limit FDA discretion by carefully spelling out procedures to be followed. This strategy is ineffective, as it has hampered the implementation of many provisions.

33. Kessler et al., "Federal Regulation," 362.

34. Food and Drug Administration, *Guidance on the Center for Devices and Radiological Health's Premarket Notification and Review Program* (Department of Health and Human Services, 1986).

35. Deborah B. Citrin, "Extracorporeal Shock-wave Lithotripsy," *Spectrum* (Arthur D. Little Decision Resources, August 1987): 2:85–88.

36. Alan N. G. Barkun and Thierry Ponchon, "Extracorporeal Biliary Lithotripsy: Review of Experimental Studies and a Clinical Update," *Annals of Internal Medicine* 112 (15 January 1990): 126–137, 126.

37. Gary M. Stephenson and Greg Freiherr, "High-Tech Attack: How Lithotripters Chip Away Stones," *Healthweek,* 4 December 1989, 25.

38. Federal payment policies were not critically important here because only a small percentage of kidney stone patients are covered by Medicare. Thus, the regulatory issues can be seen clearly.

39. For data on the industry, see *Biomedical Business International* 11 (15 July 1988): 99–101.

40. Miles Weiss and Greg Freiherr, "Romancing the Market for Stones," *Healthweek,* 4 December 1989, 18–20.

41. Tim Brightbill, "Gallstone Lithotripsy Suffers FDA Setback," *Healthweek,* 4 December 1989, 25–26. For a more scientific discussion of gallstone, or biliary, lithotripsy, see Michael Sackmann et al., "Shockwave Lithotripsy of Gallbladder Stones: The First 175 Patients," *New England Journal of Medicine* 318 (18 February 1988): 393–397. See also Barkun and Ponchon, "Extracorporeal Biliary."

42. Brightbill, 25–26.

43. Ron Winslow, "Costly Shock-wave Machines Fare Poorly on Gallstones, Disappointing Hospitals," *Wall Street Journal,* 9 February 1990, B1, B6.

44. For a complete discussion of the post-1983 Medicare coverage process, see chapter 7.

45. House Subcommittee on Health and the Environment, statement of Charles A. Bowsher, comptroller general, *Medical Devices: The Public Health at Risk,* 6 November 1989.

46. Senate Committee on Governmental Affairs, *Report to the Chairman: Early Warning of Problems Is Hampered by Severe Underreporting* (Washington, D.C.: General Accounting Office, December 1986).

47. Final Rule, 49 *Federal Register* 36326–36351 (14 September 1984).

48. Office of Management and Budget Symposium, March 1986.

49. *Medical Device Recalls* (Washington, D.C.: General Accounting Office, August 1989).

50. House Subcommittee on Health and the Environment, Committee on Energy and Commerce, statement of Gerald Sikorski and testimony of Michael B. Davis, Sr., and Cory J. Davis, 6 November 1989.

51. House Subcommittee on Health and the Environment, testimony of Charles Bowsher, *Medical Devices,* 13–15.

52. For a discussion of this case in greater detail, see Susan Bartlett Foote, "Corporate Responsibility in a Changing Legal Environment," *California Management Review* 26 (Spring 1984): 217–228, 221.

53. Consent decree signed by Procter & Gamble and the FDA (22 September 1980).

54. U.S. Department of Health and Human Services, *A Survey of Medical Device Manufacturers,* prepared for the Bureau of Medical Devices, Food and Drug Administration by Louis Harris and Associates, no. 802005 (Washington, D.C., July 1982). This comprehensive, but

early, survey concluded that the impacts were minor, although smaller firms might feel regulatory effects more strongly than larger ones.

55. Oscar Hauptman and Edward B. Roberts, "FDA Regulation of Product Risk and the Growth of Young Biomedical Firms" (Working paper, Sloan School of Management, Massachusetts Institute of Technology, 1986).

56. Mitchell, "Dynamic Commercialization." Mitchell tried to measure regulatory effects by comparing the types of firms that introduced computed tomography (CT) scanners and nuclear magnetic resonance (NMR) imaging devices. CT diffusion preceded the 1976 law and NMR was introduced subsequently. He hypothesizes that if there were more start-up companies in computer homographics than in magnetic resonance imaging, then one could conclude that there was a regulation induced bias. His data indicates there was no evidence of small-firm liability.

57. These issues will be pursued further in chapters 9 and 10.

CHAPTER 6

1. I use the term *personal injury law* to refer to both product liability and negligence—two different theories of liability. Technically, product liability refers to the legal theory of liability derived from strict liability, which assesses responsibility for defective products without concern for fault. Negligence, on the other hand, is a separate legal theory where liability is assessed on the basis of fault. Medical device producers, indeed all product producers, can be held liable under either theory. Both are discussed in greater detail in this chapter.

2. Plaintiffs generally sue everyone in the chain of distribution—manufacturers, wholesalers, retailers, and others. This discussion focuses on manufacturers.

3. See discussion of the FDA in chapter 5.

4. The lack of reliable data is substantial, a problem noted and discussed in two major studies of product liability trends. The Rand Corporation, Institute for Civil Justice issued a study by Terry Dungworth, *Product Liability and the Business Sector: Litigation Trends in Federal Courts,* R–3668–ICI (1989) and the General Accounting Office, Briefing Report to the Chairman, House Subcommittee on Commerce, Consumer Protection, and Competitiveness, Committee on Energy and Commerce, *Product Liability: Extent of 'Litigation Explosion' in Federal Courts Questions,* GAO–HRD–88–36BR (January 1988). Both studies focus on federal court filings because the data are more accessible than in state courts, where records are not uniform and are difficult to acquire. In

addition, corporate and insurance company records are confidential, and data about litigation costs or settlement amounts are not disclosed.

5. Traditionally, this area of law was dominated by common-law principles, that is, law that evolves through the judicial interpretation of precedents or previous court decisions. In state court, a state legislature can pass statutes that supercede the common-law principles; these statutes are then enforced by the court. In some states, such as California, there are also ballot initiatives that are voted on by the electorate. If the initiative passes, it becomes law and must be enforced by the court. Frequently, the courts are called upon to interpret unclear provisions in the statutes, which they must do in order to enforce the law.

6. These are called the *elements of the case*. The plaintiff must plead all the required elements in the complaint filed in the court and must prove them all to win. For further reading of tort law, see G. Edward White, *Tort Law in America: An Intellectual History* (New York: Oxford University Press, 1985). For a law and economics perspective, see Guido Calabresi, *The Costs of Accidents: A Legal and Economic Analysis* (New Haven: Yale University Press, 1970). For a basic primer on the rules of tort law, see Edward J. Kionka, *Torts in a Nutshell: Injuries to Persons and Property* (St. Paul, Minn.: West, 1977).

7. Jethro K. Lieberman, *The Litigious Society* (New York: Basic Books, 1981), 35.

8. For an interesting discussion of the history of American law, see Morton J. Horwitz, *The Transformation of American Law, 1780–1860* (Cambridge: Harvard University Press, 1977), especially chaps. 6–7. See also Grant Gilmore, *The Ages of American Law* (New Haven: Yale University Press, 1977); and Lawrence M. Friedman, *A History of American Law* (New York: Simon and Schuster, 1973).

9. With a circumscribed standard of care, it was difficult for the plaintiff to show that the defendant's conduct fell below the legally imposed standard of behavior. Defenses that the defendant could raise included contributory negligence (if the plaintiff contributed even in a minor way to his own injury, he would automatically lose) and assumption of risk (certain activities are assumed to be risky, and the plaintiff must bear the consequences of those risks he undertakes). A good defense protected defendants from liability.

10. For example, the law required that the plaintiff be a party to the contract in order to sue, thus spouses or children of the person who signed the contract for product purchase could not bring an action. This is called *privity of contract*. Contract remedies, or the amount of money that can be claimed, also were narrowly defined by contemporary personal injury standards.

11. For example, California eliminated the defense of contributory negligence in Li v. Yellow Cab, 13C. 3d 804 (1970). Now plaintiffs can prevail even if they contributed to their own harm, but their damages will be reduced by the percentage share that is attributed to their own behavior.

12. Although the principles vary from state to state, a product can be considered defective if its design leads to harm or if there is a failure to adequately warn the user of its risks.

13. 59 Cal. 2d 57, at 62. A few years earlier, in a dissenting opinion in Escola v. Coca Cola Bottling Co., Justice Traynor of the California Supreme Court set forth the grounds for the strict liability standard for product defects that was adopted by a large majority of jurisdictions nearly two decades later. While this dissent was largely ignored, it planted the seeds for the subsequent revolution. 24 Cal. 2d 453, 461 (1944).

14. The American Law Institute (ALI) does not make law. However, distinguished scholars have traditionally analyzed and evaluated trends in the law and compiled them in books known as *Restatements*. The *Restatements* are not binding on courts. However, they are frequently consulted by judges in the course of drafting opinions, are very influential, and are often cited by judges for support in altering common-law principles.

15. For a comprehensive discussion of the theory of product liability, see George Priest, "The Invention of Enterprise Liability: A Critical History of the Intellectual Foundations of Modern Tort Law," *Journal of Legal Studies* 14 (1985): 461–527. See also James A. Henderson and Theodore Eisenberg, "The Quiet Revolution in Products Liability: An Empirical Study of Legal Change," *UCLA Law Review* 37 (1990): 479–553.

16. What constitutes legal causation is another area fraught with controversy but is beyond the scope of our discussion. For those who want to understand the debate, see Steven Shavell, "An Analysis of Causation and the Scope of Liability in the Law of Torts," *Journal of Legal Studies* 9 (June 1980): 463–516.

17. Once again, a caveat on the reliability of data. Of the millions of insurance claims filed each year, only 2 percent are resolved through lawsuits. Less than 5 percent of the cases that are tried reach a verdict; the rest are settled. See Ivy E. Broder, "Characteristics of Million Dollar Awards: Jury Verdicts and Final Disbursements," *Justice System Journal* 11 (Winter 1986): 353. Many jury verdicts do not reflect what the plaintiff actually receives because these awards can be reduced on appeal. Jury awards are used as a benchmark for settlement amounts,

however, and do reflect broader trends. See discussion in Robert Litan, Peter Swire, and Clifford Winston, "The U.S. Liability System: Backgrounds and Trends," in Robert Litan and Clifford Winston, eds., *Liability: Perspectives and Policy* (Washington, D.C.: The Brookings Institution, 1988).

18. For a review of the principles of punitive damages, see Jane Mallor and Barry Roberts, "Punitive Damages: Toward a Principled Approach," *Hastings Law Journal* 31 (1980): 641–670. See also Richard J. Mahoney and Stephen P. Littlejohn, "Innovation on Trial: Punitive Damages Versus New Products," *Science* 246 (15 December 1989): 1395–1399.

19. See discussion in Andrew L. Frey, "Do Punitives Fit the Crime?" *National Law Journal*, 9 October 1989, 13–14.

20. See "Punitive Damages: How Much Is Too Much?" *Business Week*, 27 March 1989, 54–55.

21. Edward H. Levi, "An Introduction to Legal Reasoning," *University of Chicago Law Review* 15 (1948): 501–574.

22. Lester W. Feezer, "Tort Liability of Manufacturers and Vendors," *Minnesota Law Review* 10 (1925): 1–27.

23. William M. Landes and Richard A. Posner, *The Economic Structure of Tort Law* (Cambridge: Harvard University Press, 1987).

24. Priest, "Critical History," 463.

25. For detailed discussion of comment k, see Victor E. Schwartz, "Unavoidably Unsafe Products: Clarifying the Meaning and Policy Behind Comment K," *Washington and Lee Law Review* 42 (1985): 1139–1148, and Joseph A. Page, "Generic Product Risks: The Case Against Comment K and for Strict Tort Liability," *New York University Law Review* 58 (1983): 853–891. The California Supreme Court recently disapproved the holding in a prior case which would have conditioned the application of the exemption under certain circumstances. California came down squarely on the side of comment k. In holding that a drug manufacturer's liability for a design defect in a drug should not be measured by strict liability, the court reasoned that "because of the public interest in the development, availability, and reasonable price of drugs, the appropriate test for determining responsibility is comment k. . . . Public policy favors the development and marketing of beneficial new drugs, even though some risks, perhaps serious ones, might accompany their introduction, because drugs can save lives and reduce pain and suffering." Brown v. Superior Court, 44C 3d 1049, 245 Cal. Rptr. 412 (31 March 1988) at 1059.

26. The GAO report found that drug products, including bendectin, a morning sickness drug, DES, a synthetic hormone used to pre-

vent miscarriage, and Oraflex, an arthritis medicine, accounted for significant amounts of product liability litigation. GAO, "Product Liability," 12.

27. 90 Wash. 2d 9 (1978).

28. 648 P.2d 21 (Okla. 1982).

29. Ibid., 23.

30. 231 Cal. Rptr. 396 (1986).

31. For discussion of the Medical Device Amendments, see chapter 4. All Class I and Class II devices, as well as those entering the market under the 510k provision, do not undergo safety and efficacy screening similar to drugs. Some of these products may be limited to prescriptions or have labeling requirements imposed, however.

32. For a discussion of medical malpractice, see Patricia Danzon, *Medical Malpractice: Theory, Evidence, and Public Policy* (Cambridge: Harvard University Press, 1985).

33. Guerry R. Thornton, Jr., "Intrauterine Devices: IUD Cases May Be Product Liability or Medical Negligence," *Trial* (November 1986): 44–48, 44.

34. Duane Gingerich, ed., *Medical Product Liability: A Comprehensive Guide and Sourcebook* (New York: F & S Press, 1981), 57.

35. 638 S.W. 2d 660 (Ark. 1982).

36. David Lauter, "A New Rx for Liability," *National Law Journal* (15 August 1983), 1, 10.

37. Kathleen Doheny, "Liability Claims," *Medical Device and Diagnostic Industry* (June 1988): 58–61, quoting Jaxon White, President of Medmarc Insurance, Fairfax, Virginia.

38. Priest, "Critical History," 1582.

39. Michael Brody, "When Products Turn into Liabilities," *Fortune,* 3 March 1986, 20–24.

40. Luigi Mastroianni, Jr., Peter J. Donaldson, and Thomas T. Kane, eds., *Developing New Contraceptives: Obstacles and Opportunities* (Washington D.C.: National Academy Press, 1990).

41. Health Industry Manufacturers Association, "Product Liability Question Results" (Unpublished document, 14 October 1987). Forty-nine companies received the questionnaire, 39 responded. HIMA has two hundred member companies.

42. See Report BB (A–88), "Impact of Product Liability on the Development of New Medical Technologies" (Unpublished document of the American Medical Association, undated).

43. See discussion in chapter 4.

44. See Morton Mintz, *At Any Cost: Corporate Greed, Women, and the Dalkon Shield* (New York: Pantheon, 1985); Susan Perry and Jim Daw-

son, *Nightmare: Women and the Dalkon Shield* (New York: Macmillan, 1985); and Sheldon Engelmayer and Robert Wagman, *Lord's Justice: One Judge's Battle to Expose the Deadly Dalkon Shield IUD* (New York: Doubleday, 1985).

45. Hewitt v. A. H. Robins Co., No. 3–83–1291 (3rd Div. Minn., 21 February 1985).

46. Subrata N. Chakravarty, "Tunnel Vision," *Forbes,* 21 May 1984, 214–215.

47. *New York Times,* 22 August 1985, 36.

48. *Wall Street Journal,* 7 November 1989, A3.

49. Alan Cooper, "Way Is Cleared for Robins Trust," *National Law Journal,* 20 November 1989, 3, 30.

50. Ibid., 30.

51. Barry Meier, "Designer of Faulty Heart Valve Seeks Redemption in New Device," *New York Times Science,* 17 April 1990, B5–6.

52. By 1980, it was clear that some of the original valves that opened 60 degrees were malfunctioning. Bjork convinced Shiley that it should produce a 70 degree valve, which would offer improved flow. Shiley apparently remilled many of the 60 degree valves; these products were even more hazardous than those they replaced. None were sold in the United States, and they were removed from the world market in 1983. Approximately 4,000 overseas patients received the valves. By 1990, seventy had died. See discussion in Greg Rushford, "Pfizer's Telltale Heart Valve," *Legal Times,* 26 February 1990, 1, 10–13.

53. Michael Waldholz, "Pfizer Inc. Says Its Reserves, Insurance Are Adequate to Cover Heart Valve Suits," *Wall Street Journal,* 26 February 1990.

54. Greg Rushford, "Pfizer Fires Opening Salvo in Its Public Defense," *Legal Times,* 5 March 1990, 6.

55. A fraud claim differs from negligence. Fraud requires that the defendant misrepresented the product, knowingly with intent to induce the plaintiff to enter into the transaction. When fraud is involved, rather than simple negligence, the court has held that claims for anxiety can be heard. See Khan v. Shiley, Inc., 226 Cal. Rptr. 106 (30 January 1990).

56. *New York Times,* 20 October 1988.

CHAPTER 7

1. Lawrence D. Brown, "Introduction to a Decade of Transition," *Journal of Health Politics, Policy and Law* 11 (1986): 569–580, 571.

2. Detailed discussion of these major and complex institutional re-

organizations, such as HMOs (health maintenance organizations), capitation plans, and other forms of managed care, is beyond my scope here. For further reading, see Judith A. Hale and Mary M. Hunter, *From HMO Movement to Managed Care Industry: The Future of HMOs in a Volatile Healthcare Market* (Excelsior, Minn.: InterStudy Center for Managed Care Research, 1988); and Peter Boland, *Making Managed Healthcare Work: A Practical Guide to Strategies and Solutions* (New York: McGraw-Hill, 1991).

3. Stuart H. Altman and Richard Blendon, *Medical Technologies: The Culprit Behind Health Care Costs? Proceedings of the 1977 Sun Valley Forum on National Health* (Washington, D.C., 1979), cited in Gloria Ruby, H. David Banta, and Anne K. Burns, "Medicare Coverage, Medicare Costs and Medical Technology," *Journal of Health Politics, Policy and Law* 10 (1985): 141–155, n.2.

4. See Brown, "Introduction to a Decade," in which he establishes these helpful categorizations of cost-containment policies.

5. David S. Salkever and Thomas W. Bice, *Hospital Certificate-of-Need Controls: Impact on Investment, Costs, and Use* (Washington, D.C.: American Enterprise Institute, 1979), 3.

6. Social Security Amendments of 1972, sec. 259F(b).

7. Clark C. Havighurst, "Regulation of Health Facilities and Services by Certificate-of-Need," *Virginia Law Review* 59 (October 1973): 1143–1232.

8. Salkever and Bice, *Hospital Certificate-of-Need*, 20.

9. Much has been written on the prospective payment system. See U.S. Congress, Office of Technology Assessment, *Medicare's Prospective Payment System: Strategies for Evaluating Cost, Quality, and Medical Technology*, OTA–H–262 (Washington, D.C.: GPO, October 1985). See also Louise B. Russell, *Medicare's New Hospital Payment System: Is It Working?* (Washington, D.C.: The Brookings Institution, 1989).

10. In 1986, Congress created the Physician Payment Review Commission (PPRC) to advise it on reforms of the methods used to pay physicians under Medicare. Its guiding principle has been that payment reform should provide equitable payment to doctors, protect beneficiaries, and slow the rate of increase of Medicare expenditures. As part of Omnibus Budget Reconciliation Act of 1989 (OBRA), Congress enacted comprehensive reform of Medicare physician payments. For a detailed discussion of Medicare physician payment issues, see Physician Payment Review Commission, *Annual Report to Congress, 1990* (Washington, D.C.). The new fee schedule will not be in place until 1992 at the earliest. Its impact on medical device markets cannot be predicted at this time.

11. The law requires that ProPAC submit annual reports to Congress that contain its recommendations on updating the Medicare prospective payments and modifying the diagnosis related group (DRG) classification and weighing factors. Public Law 98–21, sec. 1886(e)(4). See, for example, Prospective Payment Assessment Commission, *Medicare Prospective Payment and the American Health Care System: Report to the Congress* (April 1985) and annual reports thereafter.

12. Senate Committee on Finance, *Hospital Capital Cost Reimbursement Under the Medicare Program,* prepared for the Congressional Research Service of the Library of Congress by Julian Pettengill, 5 November 1985. See also Ross M. Mullner, "Trends in Hospital Capital and the Prospective Payment System: Issues and Implications," in Henry P. Brehm and Ross M. Mullner, eds., *Health Care, Technology, and the Competitive Environment* (New York: Praeger, 1989).

13. Brehm and Mullner, *Health Care.*

14. 52 *Federal Register* 33168–33199 (1 September 1987).

15. Frank A. Sloan, Michael A. Morrisey, and Joseph Valvona, "Effects of the Medicare Prospective Payment System on Hospital Cost Containment: An Early Appraisal," *Milbank Quarterly* 66 (1988): 191–220.

16. Stephen K. Cooper, "ProPAC Nixes Capital Expenditure Reform Scheme," *Healthweek,* 7 May 1990, 15, 36. Any decision on the pass-through was delayed during 1990, and, regardless of the change, it would not take effect until 1992 or 1993. Erich Kirshner, "HCFA, AHA Maneuver on Medicare Capital Reimbursement," *Healthweek,* 30 July 1990, 9.

17. H. David Banta and Clyde J. Beheny, "Policy Formulation and Technology Assessment," *Milbank Memorial Fund Quarterly* 59 (1981): 445–479.

18. For a thorough overview of all the forms of technology assessment and the variety of institutions engaged in the enterprise, see the Institute of Medicine, *Assessing Medical Technologies* (Washington, D.C.: National Academy Press, 1985).

19. For a discussion of the institutional issues in technology assessment, see Foote, "Assessing Medical Technology."

20. Ibid., 69.

21. See discussion in chapter 4.

22. 54 *Federal Register* 4302–4318, 4308–4309 (30 January 1989).

23. William McGivney, "AMA Responds to HCFA's Proposed Coverage Criteria and Procedures," *American Medical Association Tech* 2 (May 1989): 4–6.

24. Cited in James G. Dickinson, ed., *Dickinson's FDA*, March 15, 1989, 9.

25. Ibid.

26. Public Law 101–239. See also Ron Geigle and Stanley B. Jones, "Outcomes Measurement: A Report from the Front," *Inquiry* 7 (1990): 7–13. For details on the new agency, see U.S. Department of Health and Human Services, *AHCPR: Purpose and Programs* (Washington, D.C.: September 1990).

27. Janet Ochs Wiener, ed., *Medicine and Health: Perspectives,* 9 October 1989, 1.

28. Eileen McCarthy, Robert Pokras, and Mary Moien, "National Trends in Lens Extraction: 1965–1984," *Journal of the American Optometric Association* 59 (January 1988): 31–35.

29. See chapter 4 for a detailed discussion of FDA regulation.

30. David M. Worthen et al., "Update Report on Intraocular Lenses," *American Academy of Ophthalmology* 88 (May 1981): 381–385; and Walter J. Stark et al., "The Role of the Food and Drug Administration in Ophthalmology: An Editorial," *Archives Ophthalmology* 104 (August 1986): 1145–1147.

31. *Biomedical Business International* 12 (17 May 1989): 70–71.

32. Milt Freudenheim, "Medicare's Curbs on Cataract Fees," *New York Times,* 15 November 1988, C2.

33. House Ways and Means Committee, *Medicare Reimbursement for Cataract Surgery 99–37,* 99th Cong. (Washington, D.C.: GPO, 1 August 1985).

34. Dwight E. M. Angell, "Cataract Surgeons Face a Critical Eye," *Healthweek,* 23 April 1990, 1, 8–9.

35. Freudenheim, "Medicare's Curbs."

36. Nancy M. Kane and Paul D. Manoukian, "The Effect of the Medicare Prospective Payment System on the Adoption of New Technology: The Case of Cochlear Implants," *New England Journal of Medicine* 321 (16 November 1989): 1378–1383.

37. Robin P. Michelson, "Cochlear Implants: Personal Perspectives," in Robert A. Schindler and Michael M. Merzenich, eds., *Cochlear Implants* (New York: Raven Press, 1985), 9–11.

38. William F. House, "A Personal Perspective on Cochlear Implants," in Schindler and Merzenich, *Cochlear Implants,* 13.

39. See the discussion in chapter 3 on an antiengineering bias at the NIH.

40. R. C. Bilger et al., "Evaluation of Subjects Presently Fitted with Implanted Auditory Prostheses," *Annals of Otolaryngology, Rhinology and Laryngology,* supplement 38 (1977) 86: 3–10. Discussed in F. Blair

Simmons, "History of Cochlear Implants in the United States: A Personal Perspective," in Schindler and Merzenich, *Cochlear Implants,* 1–7.

41. *Biomedical Business International* 8 (29 March 1985): 47–48.

42. Kane and Manoukian, "The Effect of Medicare," 1379.

43. Ibid., 1380.

44. Ibid., citing Cochlear Corporation personal communication.

45. Ibid.

CHAPTER 8

1. *Biomedical Business International* 11 (12 December 1988): 185.

2. *HIMA Focus,* November 1988, 6, citing data from U.S. Department of Commerce. (Newsletter of the Health Industry Manufacturers Association.)

3. Pacific Projects, "IMR Survey: The Medical Equipment and Health Care Services Market in Japan" (Tokyo, 1987). Pacific Projects, "Survey of Japanese Markets for Medical Equipment," vol. 1 (Tokyo, 1979).

4. Our discussion is limited to trade issues involving medical devices. For in-depth analysis of trade issues generally, see Clyde V. Prestowitz, Jr., *Trading Places: How We Allowed Japan to Take the Lead* (New York: Basic Books, 1988). For discussion of Japanese industrial organization see Chalmers Johnson, *MITI and the Japanese Miracle: The Growth of Industrial Policy 1925–1975* (Stanford: Stanford University Press, 1982); and James C. Abegglen and George Stalk, Jr., *Kaisha: The Japanese Corporation* (New York: Basic Books, 1985).

5. Vincent A. Bucci, "Japanese Import Restrictions on Medical Devices—An Overview of Recent Statutory Changes," *Food, Drug, Cosmetic Law Journal* 39 (1984): 405–410.

6. See discussion in Susan Bartlett Foote and William Mitchell, "Selling American Medical Equipment in Japan," *California Management Review* 31 (1989): 146–161, 149. See also M. H. Piscatelli, "American-Japanese Trade Impasse: The Regulation of Medical Device Imports into Japan," *Syracuse Journal of International Law and Commerce* 12 (1985): 157–169.

7. Piscatelli, "American-Japanese," 159–160.

8. U.S. and Japan MOSS Negotiating Teams, *Report on Medical Equipment and Pharmaceutical Market-Oriented, Sector-Selective (MOSS) Discussions* (Washington, D.C.: GPO, 1986).

9. Koichi Ichikawa, "Outlook for the Medical Equipment Industry Bleak in the Short Run: Brighter in the Long Run," *Business Japan,* June 1985, 71.

10. Bucci, "Japanese Import Restrictions," 407. The Japanese are not the only nation skeptical of foreign clinical test data. Indeed, the United States has its own reservations. The FDA dismisses many foreign tests as scientifically flawed or poorly inspected. Problems in reviewing foreign studies arise due to different research traditions and language barriers. See Louis Lasagna, "On Reducing Waste in Foreign Clinical Trials and Postregulation Experience," *Clinical Pharmacology and Therapeutics* 40 (1986): 369–372.

11. MOSS Negotiating Teams, *Report.*

12. William G. Mitchell and Susan Bartlett Foote, "Staying the Course: Comparative Stability of American and Japanese Firms in International Medical Equipment Markets" (Unpublished working paper, University of California, Berkeley, 1988).

13. M. Hashimoto, "Health Services in Japan," in Michael W. Raffel, ed., *Comparative Health Systems* (University Park, Penn.: Pennsylvania State University Press, 1984).

14. Pacific Projects, "IMR Survey."

15. R. Niki, "The Wide Distribution of CT Scanners in Japan," *Social Science Medicine* 21 (1985): 1131–1137.

16. Pacific Projects, "IMR Survey"; and "Drug Manufacturers Seek Greater Pricing Flexibility," *Japan Economic Journal* 30 (May 1987): 21.

17. For interesting discussions of these issues, see John Steslicke, *Doctors in Politics: The Political Life of the Japan Medical Association* (New York: Praeger, 1973); and Emiko Ohnuki-Tierney, *Illness and Culture in Japan: An Anthropological View* (Cambridge: Cambridge University Press, 1984).

18. U.S. Department of Commerce, International Trade Administration, *U.S. Imports of Medical Equipment, 1983–1986* (Unpublished report, 1987).

19. Japanese firms fear that their corporate images would be damaged if patient deaths were to be associated with products bearing their names. There is also a cultural inhibition against introducing artificial devices into the body. American companies have been more willing to advocate implants than have Japanese firms; doctors have been receptive because of the medical and financial benefits of implants.

20. Michael Rappa, "Capital Financing Strategies of the Japanese Semiconductor Industry," *California Management Review* 27 (Winter 1985): 85–99.

21. For a detailed discussion of successful organizational strategies in Japan, see Foote and Mitchell, "Selling American Medical Equipment," 153–158.

22. Ibid.

23. Current European Community members include the United Kingdom, Greece, Ireland, the Netherlands, Belgium, Luxembourg, Denmark, Germany, Italy, Spain, Portugal, and France.

24. *Biomedical Business International* 9 (12 December 1988): 185.

25. Article 155, Treaty of Rome (25 March 1957).

26. For an excellent summary of the organization of the EC, see Oppenheimer, Wolff, & Donnelly, "An Overview of the European Community's 1992 Program" (Prepared for the Health Industry Manufacturers Association, 9 November 1988).

27. International Business Communications, "European Regulation of Medical Devices and Surgical Products, including Electromedical Devices" (Conference materials, New Orleans, 14–15 November 1988), 13.

28. European Confederation of Medical Suppliers Associations (EUCOMED), "Regulation of Medical Devices and Surgical Products in Europe: How to Achieve Harmonisation" (Conference proceedings, Brussels, 9–10 March 1987), 293.

29. White paper from the Commission to the European Council, 14 June 1985.

30. Kshitij Mohan, "EC Directives Don't Spell Harmony Yet," *Medical Device and Diagnostic Industry* 12 (June 1990): 10–12.

31. William W. Lowrance, *Of Acceptable Risk: Science and the Determination of Safety* (Los Altos, Calif.: William Kauffman, 1976).

32. Economists Advisory Group, "The 'Cost of Non-Europe' in the Pharmaceutical Industry," executive summary, January 1988, cited in Oppenheimer, Wolff, and Donnelly, "An Overview," 15.

33. Ibid.

34. For an interesting discussion of voluntary and regulatory standard setting in the United States, see Ross Cheit, *Setting Safety Standards: Regulation in the Public and Private Sectors* (Berkeley: University of California Press, 1990).

35. Gary Stephenson, "International Standards: Harmonizing to a European Tune," *Medical Device and Diagnostic Industry* 12 (June 1990): 97–99.

36. "Reshaping Europe: 1992 and Beyond," *Business Week,* 12 December 1988, 48–73.

37. Stephenson, "International Standards," 98.

38. Teh-wei Hu, "Diffusion of Western Medical Technology in China Since the Economic Reform," *International Journal of Technology Assessment in Health Care* (1988): 345–358. This excellent article provides the background for the discussion that follows.

39. U.S. Department of Commerce, Coopers & Lybrand Report, cited in *Biomedical Business International* 12 (16 January 1989): 12–13.

40. Hu, "Diffusion," 353.

CHAPTER 9

1. The epigraph for part 3 is from Stephan Tanneberger, "When Must a New Approach to Treatment Be Introduced?" *International Journal of Technology Assessment in Health Care* 4 (1988), 113.

2. Fred Dotzler and John Reher, "What Market Segments Attract Venture Capital Firms," *Medical Device and Diagnostic Industry* 11 (September 1989): 84–86.

3. See the discussion of the impact of NIH disapproval on cochlear implants in chapter 7.

4. Interview with Dr. Peer Portnor, December 1988.

5. Spyros Andreopoulos, "A Helper for the Ailing Heart," *Stanford Medicine* (Fall 1986): 6–9.

6. Interview with Dr. Peer Portnor.

7. The Population Council, news release, 28 October 1987.

8. Don Colburn, "Informed Consent Eases the Return of IUDs," *Washington Post,* 10 November 1987, 7.

9. "Progestasert: Intrauterine Progesterone Contraceptive System Patient Information" (Alza Corporation, 1986). Interview with Peter Carpenter, vice president of Alza Corporation, January 1987.

10. "Careful Patient Selection Allows for Return of Copper IUD to U.S. Market," *American College of Obstetrics and Gynecology* 32 (January 1988): 1, 11.

11. Gary Stephenson and Greg Freiherr, "Products that Won Big in 1987," *Medical Device and Diagnostic Industry* 10 (July 1988): 26, n. 13.

12. For an interesting British view of the NIH and its political environment, see Richard Smith, "Glimpses of the National Institutes of Health: Funding and Structure," *British Medical Journal* 296 (27 February 1988): 631–634. Specific programs often are introduced because of the personal interest of particular congressional members. In 1988, an amendment to create a new institute on deafness was offered by Tom Harkin, who has a deaf brother and is chair of the House Subcommittee on the Handicapped. Opponents argued against proliferation of institute-level components within the NIH.

13. Ibid.

14. Senate Subcommittee on Labor, Health and Human Services, Education and Related Agencies, Committee on Appropriations.

Statement of Frank E. Samuel, Jr., president, Health Industry Manufacturers Association, on the 1989 fiscal year budget request of the National Institutes of Health, 24 May 1988.

15. Henry Waxman is chair of the Subcommittee on Health and the Environment (part of the House Committee on Energy and Commerce). John Dingell is chair of the House Committee on Energy and Commerce and heads the Subcommittee on Oversight and Investigations.

16. *Congressional Record,* 4 August 1989, E 2830.

17. Ibid., E 2815.

18. See discussion in chapter 5.

19. In 1989, a scandal erupted in the generic drug industry when evidence that some firms had bribed FDA regulators with illegal gratuities. Two other firms admitted giving the FDA falsified data on their products. See Bruce Ingersoll and Gregory Stricharchuk, "Generic-Drug Scandal at the FDA Is Linked to Deregulation Drive," *Wall Street Journal,* 13 September 1989, 1, 10. See also Malcolm Gladwell, "A Few Bad Generic Drugs Can Spoil the Whole Industry," *Washington Post National Weekly Edition,* 21–27 August 1989, 31. See also American Enterprise Institute, *Proposals for Reform of Drug Regulation Law, Legislative Analysis,* no. 8 (Washington, D.C.: 1979).

It is ironic that consumer groups have generally supported these efforts until the AIDS crisis. AIDS activists have excoriated the FDA for being too slow in approving drugs for potentially lifesaving purposes, demanding less, not more, premarket scrutiny. No such forces are at work on the device side, so traditional congressional demands for greater safety have been unchallenged.

20. *Healthweek,* 10 November 1988, 7.

21. House Committee on Energy and Commerce, *Report to Accompany H.R. 3095, H. Rept. 101–808,* 101st Cong., 2d sess. (5 October 1990). See also Senate Committee on Labor and Human Resources, *Report to Accompany S. 3006, S. Rept. 101–513,* 101st Cong., 2d sess. (9 October 1990).

22. The Rand Corporation, Institute for Civil Justice, *Tort Policy Working Report,* February 1986.

23. Other studies have challenged these findings. The General Accounting Office issued a report in 1988 (*Product Liability: Extent of Litigation Explosion in Federal Courts Questioned*) that found that, at least in federal court filings, most claims related to asbestos (40 percent of growth), the Dalkon Shield (12 percent), and bendectin (5 percent).

24. Sheila R. Shulman, "Tort Reform Activities in the United

States," in Sheila R. Shulman and Louis Lasagna, eds., *Trends in Product Liability Law and No-Fault Compensation for Drug-Induced Injuries* (Boston: Center for the Study of Drug Development, 1990), 46–49.

25. Ibid., citing *An Act Concerning Product Liability and Punitives Damages*, State of New Jersey, chap. 197, laws of 1987, 47.

26. Presumptions in this context mean a rule of law in which the court will draw a particular inference from a particular fact unless and until the truth of such inference is disproved. This means that the presumption works in favor of the defendant, assuming that there has been adequate warning, unless the plaintiff proves otherwise.

27. S. 1400, the Product Liability Reform Act, was introduced in the Senate in July 1989. Congressional hearings on the measure got underway in January 1990. Attempts to pass similar legislation go back ten years. There were four medical malpractice bills pending in Congress in the summer of 1991, including S. 1386, introduced by Senators Durenberger, Danforth, and McCain, which includes a government standards defense for drugs and medical devices.

28. For a discussion of the Supreme Court's recent decisions involving review of punitive damages in a variety of contexts, see Andrew Frey, "Do Punitives Fit the Crime?" *National Law Journal,* 9 October 1989, 13–14.

29. It is ironic that before the advent of the prospective payment system, Medicare was a boon to producers of products used primarily by beneficiaries. Now, with cost containment, a market dominated by Medicare can be the most difficult.

30. Of course, predictions are always risky in the health care field. If the PSS completely breaks down, hospitals become bankrupt in large numbers or new public health crises erupt, the system could fail, and a new one could be imposed. Any new system would inevitably include some decision-making mechanism for technology adoption and diffusion, however. Cost controls are not likely to go away no matter what kind of public payment system is adopted.

31. The position of the pharmaceutical industry could change in the future given proposals to include drugs within the Medicare coverage.

32. Surveys indicate considerable ambivalence among consumers. In general, they say that cost control is necessary, but do not personally want to see any limitations on access to all forms of high-tech care.

33. Ben F. Small, "Gaffing at a Thing Called Cause: Medico-Legal Conflicts in the Concept of Causation," *Texas Law Review* 31 (1953): 630–659, 655.

34. Compliance with FDA regulations would occur, however, if the government standards defense were widely imposed.

35. Much of this discussion is relevant to policy reform for pharmaceuticals as well.

36. See Foote, "Product Liability." The proposal, in brief, is to expand FDA authority so that it can compensate for device related injuries and can refer cases of fraud to the courts to impose a punitive function. The producer would benefit from compliance with the FDA. Only those who fail to comply would face judicial remedies. Such a system could be extended to all medical technologies, including pharmaceuticals, and could also encompass medical malpractice concerns.

37. Aspects of the National Childhood Vaccine Injury Compensation Program are similar. See U.S. Congress, *Hearings before the Senate Committee on Labor and Human Resources,* 98th Cong., 1st sess., 1984, S. Rept. 98–1060. In that program, plaintiffs injured by certain vaccines can choose a traditional product liability remedy, with some limitations, or an expedited administrative proceeding. For an interesting proposal, see The Keystone Center, "Keystone AIDS Vaccine Liability Project Final Report" (Keystone, Colo.: Keystone Center, May 1990).

38. See Danzon, *Medical Malpractice.* See also the work of Steven Sugarman critiquing the liability system, in particular, "Doing Away with Tort Law," *California Law Review* 73 (May 1985): 555–664.

39. The Interagency Task Force on Products Liability estimated that 40 percent of premiums go for underwriting expenses and profit and 20 percent of premiums go for loss-adjustment expenses; that leaves only forty cents of every premium available to compensate victims. See also Sugarman, "Doing Away," 591–600.

40. Public Law 98–369.

41. Cardiac Pacemaker Registry, 51 *Federal Register* 16792–16799 (6 May 1986).

42. Final Rule, Cardiac Pacemaker Registry, 52 *Federal Register* 27756–27765 (23 July 1987).

43. Sources have described such turf wars between the National Cancer Institute and the FDA. However, in the context of AIDS research, an emergency situation, the NCI and the FDA cooperated in designing research and approval mechanisms for new drugs.

44. *Biomedical Business International* 12 (20 June 1989): 84.

CHAPTER 10

1. Opening quote from Oliver Sacks, *Awakenings* (New York: Harper Collins, 1990), 226.

2. Daniel Callahan, *What Kind of Life: The Limits of Medical Progress* (New York: Simon and Schuster, 1990), 101.

3. Richard M. Neustadt, *Presidential Power* (New York: John Wiley, 1976), 101.

4. Callahan, *What Kind of Life,* 97.

Index

A. H. Robins Company, 118, 119–20,
150–51, 156
Abbott Laboratories, 188
Abrams, Albert, 36
Academic journals, 59–60
Acidimeter, 32
Activitrax, 109
Acuson, 213–14
Acute care facilities, 87
Agency for Health Care Policy and Re-
search (AHCPR), 169
Agriculture Appropriations Act, 42
AIDS (acquired immune deficiency syn-
drome), 229, 232–33, 235, 273n.19,
275n.37
Airco v. Simmons First National Bank,
147–48
Alza Corporation, 14–15, 156, 157, 210
AMA (American Medical Association),
87–88, 149, 168
American College of Obstetricians and
Gynecologists (ACOG), 169
American Law Institute (ALI), 141,
262n.14
American Medical Association (AMA),
87–88, 149, 168
American Science and Engineering
(AS&E), 104
American Telephone and Telegraph
(AT&T), 29–30
AMP v. Gardner, 116
Antibiotic disk, 117
Arkansas Supreme Court, 148
Artificial heart, 61, 62
Artificial Heart Program (AHP), 21,
62–65, 81, 205–7, 233, 250n.19
Artificial kidney, 85, 100
Artificial kidney machine, 22, 99–102
AT&T (American Telephone and Tele-
graph), 29–30
AutoMicrobic System (AMS), 68
Automobile industry, 8, 241–42n.12
AZT (zidovudine), 14

Baker, Russell, 26
Bakken, Earl, 107
Battery technology, 106
Baxter, Donald, 51
Baxter Travenol, 51, 102

Bayh-Dole Patent and Trademark
Amendments, 79
Beckman, Arnold, 32–33
Beckman Instruments, 32–33, 49–51
Beem, John R., 63
Beutel, Albert, 108
Biliary lithotripsy, 129
Biologics Control Act, 39
Biomedical research: engineering's re-
lationship with, 29, 64, 71; govern-
ment support of, 40, 56–58, 77, 84,
204, 217; and medical devices, 81;
and medical practice, 28–29. *See also*
Research
Bjork-Shiley Convexo-Concave heart
valve, 152, 154
Bjork, Viking O., 152
"Boiling soup" concept, 57
Brandeis, Louis Dembitz, 237
Buick Motor Company, 140
Bush, George, 219

California Supreme Court, 141
Callahan, Daniel, 235–36, 237
Campbell, W. G., 43
Capital-cost pass-through, 164–65
Capital expenditures, 91–92, 105, 164,
165
Cardiac Pacemaker (CPI), 108
Cardiac pacemakers. *See* Pacemakers
Cardiology, 61–62, 106
Cardozo, Benjamin, 140
Cataracts, 171–72, 173
Census of Manufactures, 11, 37
Center for Devices and Radiological
Health (CDRH), 231
Centers for Disease Control (CDC),
135
Cerebellar stimulator, 124, 258n.30
Certificate of Need (CON) programs,
23, 160, 161, 162, 215
Chardack, William, 107
China, 197–99, 200; Ministry of
Health, 198, 199; National Bureau
of Medical and Pharmaceutical
Management, 198; Price Bureau,
199
China Medical Instrument Corpora-
tion, 198

Compositor: Keystone Typesetting, Inc.
Text: 11/13 Baskerville
Display: Baskerville
Printer and Binder Maple-Vail Book Mfg. Group